Sheena Byrom was born and brought up in north-west
England

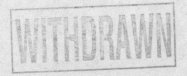

years. She has ntly
taken ormal child
bir ried with
four children, one whom has followed her mother's
footsteps in becoming a midwife lecturer.

Catching Babies

Sheena Byrom

with Charlotte Ward

headline

First published in 2011
by HEADLINE PUBLISHING GROUP

1

Cataloguing in Publication Data is available from the British Library

ISBN 978 0 7553 6272 1

Typeset in Dante by Avon DataSet Ltd,
Bidford-on-Avon, Warwickshire

Printed and bound by
CPI Group (UK) Ltd, Croydon, CR0 4YY

Headline's policy is to use papers that are natural, renewable and
recyclable products and made from wood grown in sustainable forests.
The logging and manufacturing processes are expected to conform to the
environmental regulations of the country of origin.

HEADLINE PUBLISHING GROUP
An Hachette UK Company
338 Euston Road
London NW1 3BH

www.headline.co.uk
www.hachette.co.uk

This book is dedicated to women. My career has high-lighted over and over again the wonders and resilience of females, and the fact that they 'hold up the world'. For me, the greatest woman was my mother, Kathleen Murray. Kathleen gave birth to five girls, all destined to carry on her legacy. For the women born to my sisters, and the daughters of the sons, this small section of our family history is for you, told and written with you in mind.

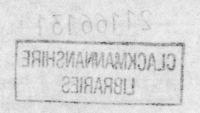
All the events portrayed in this book are true. However, in order to protect confidentiality, certain names, dates, locations and other details have been changed. The author is grateful to all those who gave their consent to their stories being told in this book.

Prologue

Waking with a jolt, I heard the telephone ringing.

As always my heart raced as my eyes sprang open. Next to me in bed my husband Paul stirred but was clearly still out for the count. By now he was well used to the 'bat phone' going off in the middle of the night.

As the shrill ring continued I jumped out of bed and grabbed the telephone receiver.

'Hi,' I croaked, clearing my throat.

'Sheena, it's Angela.' My colleague's voice filtered down the line. 'Jan is in labour. Are you still OK to come and assist?'

'Give me ten minutes,' I replied. Then hanging up the phone, I pulled off my nightie and quickly changed into my work clothes.

Grabbing my bag I raced to the door, stopping moment-arily to glance into my daughter Olivia's bedroom. As I suspected she was tucked up peacefully, in a deep slumber.

Racing out the door and into the dark I headed off down the road and within minutes found myself outside Jan's semi-detached home.

Angela met me at the door. 'Thanks, Sheena,' she smiled.

'No problem,' I beamed back, the excitement of another impending birth now racing through my veins.

Inside the house I found Jan, a friendly woman in her early thirties, ready in her birthing pool. This was Jan's fourth baby and she'd specifically requested a water birth. Her husband Joe was there and her three elder children were sat on the sofa having been allowed to stay up to meet their new sibling.

The room had dimmed lighting and the atmosphere was calm. There was a gentle lapping sound as Jan swayed in the water while, in the background, James Taylor played quietly on the stereo.

As Jan worked through her contractions, her eyes almost trance-like, Angela and I sat on the floor and watched, getting up to examine her from time to time.

Finally, when Jan was ready to give birth, we positioned ourselves nearer, watching in awe as slowly but surely she pushed her baby out. With one last mighty effort she finally freed her daughter into the water and scooped her up to the surface. I held my breath as Jan held her little girl gently in her hands, examining her features for the very first time with a look of pure love and wonder. Baby Susan had arrived in the world.

After we'd checked the baby over and delivered the placenta, Angela and I settled Jan down to breastfeed. Sitting nearby we smiled with encouragement at the sweet sound of baby Susan's little contented noises as she enjoyed her very first feed.

As I watched this special moment between mother and daughter – the circle of life unfolding before me – I thought for a moment about all the other women I'd met and helped to give birth.

I would never fail to be amazed by the strength of mothers pushing with all their might to bring their babies into the world. Likewise the sheer joy of birth and seeing a new life starting out in the world would always enthrall me. I feel uniquely privileged to be able to witness this miracle on an almost daily basis and to be able to assist women during one of the most important days of their lives. It is something I feel I was born to do.

Chapter 1

Lying in a huge bed, I scanned the open ward in front of me, eager to catch a glimpse of my favourite nurse.

I wriggled my toes under my white bedsheets, watching as flashes of blue went past me – nurses dashing from patient to patient, carrying bedpans and trays.

Then at last I spotted Nurse Ferris, a tall woman with dark-brown hair tied up in a bun and, best of all, a lovely smile on her face. As she walked towards me it just made my ten-year-old heart soar.

Here was the one nurse who, during my two-week stint in hospital, had always stopped to chat and smile at me, and comforted me when I was scared.

It was her alone who helped to ease the anxious feeling in my tummy as I faced each day on Ward Seven and who, unbeknown to her, would have a great influence on me when some eight years later I would become a nurse myself.

When I qualified as a nurse and later as a midwife, I would always think back to those early years when I'd been blighted by a spleen condition and endured two childhood stints in hospital.

My first experience of hospital was in 1963 when, aged

just eight, I'd suffered repeat bouts of nausea. I'd been feeling sick at school and – because both my mother and the eldest of my four sisters, Lynne, had suffered enlarged spleens and had had surgery to remove them – it looked highly likely that I had the same problem.

I was duly taken to see a paediatrician called Dr Moss, who was scarily grave, didn't speak to me directly and poked my stomach. A lot.

His conclusion was that I should go into hospital for some tests to confirm my condition and examine how the sickness was affecting me. On his advice a date was arranged for me to be admitted to Queens Park Hospital in Blackburn, on the CH3 ward, which was specifically for children with 'medical' problems.

On the day I was admitted I left home on my own in an ambulance, my lip wobbling as I bid Mum goodbye and climbed into the back. As the doors shut behind me I tried to remember Mum's advice.

'There will be other children there who are sick,' she warned. 'But you mustn't worry as you will be fine.'

I'd never been separated from my parents before and the prospect of being apart from them for a week seemed like an eternity.

CH3 was a prefabricated structure situated on the edge of the hospital grounds, away from the other buildings. It felt more like a hut and there were partitioned areas within the ward to separate children of different ages. It all seemed very unwelcoming and clinical, and I can distinctly remember its strange, fusty, disinfectant smell. From then on it was a smell I immediately associated with illness and injections.

From the off I was terrified and felt incredibly homesick. My anxiety was only enhanced by the fact that some of the other children were obviously much sicker than me. One was in a wheelchair and some were bed bound. I'd never seen illness to that degree.

I had numerous blood tests that were sprung on me with no warning – unlike today where procedures are routinely explained – and I never knew if they were going to be repeated. Whenever a nurse or doctor came near me I worried that I would have to have yet another needle put in my arm.

There was a room attached to the ward where we went for school lessons. This broke the days up as they were long with little to do. I don't remember any toys or games and of course visitors were scarce. Although I did not know it at the time, this was partly because of the hospital regime and partly because my parents couldn't get to the hospital easily.

I was desperate to go home and asked constantly when that would be. When the time finally came to be discharged, I was bursting with excitement. But it wasn't to be my last stay on a hospital ward.

During my stay in hospital I'd been diagnosed with a condition called acholuric jaundice. Although I didn't have any of the symptoms of jaundice, one of the side effects was having an enlarged spleen, so it was decided I should have it removed. So in 1965, aged ten, I returned to hospital to have a splenectomy. This time I would be in for two whole weeks.

When Mum explained to me that I needed an operation, I didn't really understand the implications. After all, my sister and mum had had the same operation and they were fine.

'It will help you to stop feeling sick all the time,' Mum assured me, so when the time came for me to go back into hospital I did my best to be brave.

This time I was admitted to Ward Eight at Blackburn Royal Infirmary, a huge room known as a 'Nightingale Ward', in which the cots and beds are situated around the edges of the room, and the desk for the nurses stands in the middle. I learned later that this layout was masterminded by Florence Nightingale, who – it is said – wanted to make sure she could see everyone at one glance.

I was intimidated by the sheer size of the room, and the bed to which I was allocated had an iron headboard and seemed intimidatingly high and bare. This ward was for children who were recovering from surgery or needed an operation and I remember some were quite sick. It seemed like the babies were always crying. Of course when I think about this now it makes me feel quite sad, as the babies were probably crying for their parents – who of course were absent most of the time.

My stark memories of this time have never left me and no doubt helped me when I went on to be a nurse myself. When you've been a patient you can really empathise with what other people might be going through. You've had an insight into the stress, anxiety and sense of uncertainty. Years later I could always take myself back to that feeling of being a frightened little girl in an alien place and I tried to use that experience to understand how patients in my care might be feeling.

Both times I was in hospital the wards were run like clockwork with rigid routines. At 6 a.m. sharp all the lights went on and temperatures were taken. As you'd expect, most of the children were asleep when this happened and when the lights came on, the crying started.

After being momentarily blinded by the bright and harsh lights, I would feel dazed as I sleepily struggled to remember where I was. Then through my squinting eyes I would see a hand coming towards me with a thermometer that was swiftly placed in my mouth. I wanted more than anything to go back to sleep but with all the noise – and breakfast being served on the dot at 7 a.m. – there was no chance.

I realised later that this routine was carried out so that the night staff could get all the children sorted before shift handover. It may have been 'orderly' but it was a very regimented process and certainly made me, as a child, feel even more homesick. When, years later, I would wake patients up on the wards I would always try to be gentle and smile in the hope that it would help to put them at ease.

Apart from Nurse Ferris I don't remember the nurses being particularly warm. When I look back now I can see they were probably concerned with getting on with their work, but as a child I didn't rationalise that. I missed my parents, especially my mum, who was very tactile and loving.

At home I felt Mum's love constantly and it was the hugs, kisses and squeezes that I missed the most. The nurses didn't help me to feel safe or happy in that way. They weren't bad or cruel; they just didn't seem interested.

Nurse Ferris, on the other hand, had an amazing effect

on me. I thought she was really pretty but it was her gentleness and kindness that made her special.

'You're going to be just fine, Sheena,' she'd tell me and I'd see her going around the ward reassuring the other youngsters too.

My bed was located at the top of the ward, furthest away from the entrance. There was a radio speaker fastened to the wall quite high up, where the local radio blared out from early morning to evening.

I'd been admitted to Ward Eight on a Saturday, two days before my operation, and I can remember lying on my bed with a real feeling of dread.

During the weekend the Mamas and the Papas' hit 'Monday, Monday' was playing from the speakers above my head. Monday was the day of my operation and when I heard the lyrics 'can't trust that day', I felt a cold chill. Even when I hear that song now nearly forty-five years later it takes me back to that sense of foreboding in a heartbeat. I really didn't know what was going to happen when Monday came round.

But the day dawned, and off I went. My favourite nurse wasn't on that morning, as she was on a day off. I was sick with fear. It was such a shocking feeling when the nurse came to my bed and asked me to put on a gown. She put a cap on my head and gave me an injection – there was no explanation but it made me feel drowsy, which helped.

As they wheeled me off to the theatre my mouth was dry and I wanted to cry. Down the old corridors I went, lying flat on a trolley being pushed by a porter dressed in white. When I arrived in theatre I looked around the place fearfully until a male doctor told me I was going to sleep. He put a needle in my arm, and in a split second I was out cold.

The next thing I knew I was waking up from the operation and – joy of joys – aware my lovely mum was next to me holding my hand! I had the side of a cot up on my bed to stop me from falling out and she was leaning over it. She was smiling, and I felt safe.

There was no pain, I just felt sleepy. Up until that point I hadn't seen my parents since they'd dropped me off. Yet I hadn't seen much of anyone else's parents either, except a few at visiting time.

Some children didn't have any visitors at all. I discovered when I became a nurse almost a decade later that this was still the case, although it was changing. Parents were generally perceived as problematic; they might get in the way, and fussing over children seemed to be frowned upon in those days. There was a kind of certainty that the medical profession knew best, and parents (including mine) gave their children to the doctor's care with full acceptance that it was the right thing to do. Perhaps the hospital staff also felt that the presence of parents would cause the children to be upset by their comings and goings. I never asked my mum whether she wanted to be there or not. But it can't have been easy for her either. When my daughter Olivia went into hospital aged three I can remember being frantic with worry and I never left her side. I slept on a chair all night, and noticed other parents doing the same. But that would never have happened when I was a child. Mum left at some stage, whilst I was still asleep, leaving a message with a nurse to tell me one of my sisters would come that evening.

As good as Mum's word, Lynne, my eldest sister arrived with a wonderful gift for me: a doll who looked just like Emma Peel, a character in the popular TV show *The Avengers*! I was absolutely thrilled, and even though I couldn't sit up or keep my eyes open for long, I felt very happy.

However, for the rest of my stay I was back in the ward routine, homesick and now feeling pretty sore to boot. I walked with a bent back, guarding my stomach. I was now sporting a huge scar on my abdomen and hated it being dressed, as I didn't want to look at it. Of course, Nurse Ferris came on duty frequently and helped me to feel better. She'd sit with me, touch my arm, sort my pillows and make me feel good. I was quite a shy child and it took me a while to pluck up the courage to ask for things but she'd sit down next to me and talk to me until I found my voice. Her approach and manner were wonderful and when she smiled I felt instantly comforted.

When I became a nurse myself eight years later I always tried to be like Nurse Ferris. I remembered how her smile made me feel, and always tried to do the same when working on the wards. I think it paid off too, as on one of my first ward placements at Queens Park Hospital one of the elderly gentlemen I was caring for gave me a wonderful compliment.

'When will you be on again?' he asked.

'Tomorrow morning,' I told him brightly.

'I'm really glad,' he said. 'All the patients like it when

you are on. You've got a lovely smile.' I was really delighted to think that I'd had my own Nurse Ferris effect on a patient.

Later in my career I helped to lead an educational programme about the importance of caring and connecting with patients within a health-care setting. Almost all individuals who go to hospital either as a patient or a relative will have some form of anxiety and our message to nurses and other healthcare professionals was that you should never underestimate the importance of smiling as a fundamental part of caring.

Apart from my two operations my childhood was quite uneventful, although to my great blessing, it was full of love and security. I was the youngest daughter of five girls and the story goes that my father wanted a boy – but was nonetheless happy when he saw me.

One close neighbour, Pat, often recounted the tale of the time Dad came round the corner of our cul-de-sac and proudly announced, 'It's another girl!' I can never remember feeling that my parents were disappointed with my gender. I just remember happy days, full of girls and, of course, being the youngest of five sisters has been such an influence on my life, and what I ended up doing.

My mother Kathleen was gentle and loving though she could be feisty when she needed to be. She was the matriarch of our family and had strong moral values, clearly imparting to us what was right and wrong.

She'd been one of nine children, born in Lancashire to working-class parents, Richard (Dick) and Gertrude. The nine children were quite close all through their lives, and even though Uncle Tom was killed just after the Second World War, Betty his wife and Pam his only child stayed in touch with the brood. Mum's parents lived with us for a while in one of our downstairs rooms, and as a child I remember many visits from Mum's siblings – especially Uncle Bill as he always used to slip a shilling into my hand!

Aunty Pat was the youngest of Mum's family. She was a midwife and single, so able to spend her days off helping Mum with my grandparents – and sorting us out too! She was quite strict and when she was babysitting she would instruct us to clean the house, and thoroughly at that. But she was a great support to Mum, and to us too.

Our house was located on a small cul-de-sac of about twelve houses on a council estate in Clitheroe, a thriving market town in rural Lancashire. The estate was always buzzing with life, and everyone seemed to know each other and look out for one another. There was a real community spirit and a sense of trust and belonging.

However, it's strange how some of your perceptions as a child are quite different from reality. I was to learn in later years that my parents, like many others, struggled to make ends meet, yet I was oblivious and felt lucky to live in a 'big' house (it now seems small!) with a garden and plenty of neighbouring children and sisters to play with. It's only now I look back that I can see we were quite poor: we didn't even have a carpet or central heating. My children now look at me disbelievingly when I tell them about the ice inside the windows, and how we used to huddle round the coal fire to get warm.

My dad James (christened Seamus) was proudly Irish and

had come to England as a nineteen-year-old to find work and hopefully start a new life. He'd been born in a small village called Largan near Sligo in the west of Ireland as the second child to Michael and Bridget Murray.

Sadly, both Dad and his older sister Agnes (christened Bridget) were to have a difficult childhood: their mother died when they were very young, and their father travelled to America to try to make a living but never came back. As a result, Dad and Aunty Agnes were cared for by their grandparents and cousins, and were apparently very unhappy. Eventually Agnes moved to Yorkshire after securing a position as housekeeper to a Catholic priest, and Dad soon followed. With his sister's help he found manual work close by in Clitheroe, building roads.

It wasn't long before Dad – dark and handsome, with his lovely Irish lilt – captured Mum's attention at a local dance. She too was a head-turner, with her fair hair and blue eyes. The couple courted and soon announced their engagement.

Lynne was born first. Then Anne, Susan and Eileen followed over the next ten years. I was born when Lynne was thirteen. I remember all my sisters being around for some of my childhood, but the elder members moved on as I grew up.

Lynne, to everyone's excitement, married a professional footballer called Chris Simms, while Anne went to be a nurse in Burnley. Susan left shortly afterwards, moving to Liverpool to train to be a teacher. While my sisters never returned to live at home we remained incredibly close.

It was Eileen who played the largest part in my life. Eileen is five years older than me and has always been a huge influence. We spent hours together in our childhood and still do, and I always looked to my elder sister for guidance – and fun!

In my ninth year, my parents were given the opportunity to buy a rundown shop located on the corner terrace of a street called St Hubert's Road in Great Harwood. With Mum's skills as a trained baker and confectioner, they decided to open a bakery business with the aim of raising their standard of living. Mum, Dad, Eileen and I moved above the shop, along with Grandad Dick, who came with us to live upstairs in one of the bedrooms.

The excitement was uncontainable as Eileen and I planned how many cakes we would be able to eat, all for free. But little did we know how much our blissful, relaxed family life was about to change.

It transpired that running a family business was to have a major impact on my parents and on our day-to-day routines. The times of our meals changed, we had no dining room table on which to eat, and any free time was spent washing up baking equipment and serving in the shop.

I really didn't like it. Mum's working day started at 5 a.m. when she prepared the bread mix, so she was always tired and most nights she needed to go to bed at 8 p.m. While Dad also got up at the crack of dawn to help her, he would soon have to go off to work. Consequently Eileen and I had to help as much as we could, before and after school. Complaining wasn't allowed.

We also had to learn to live with the mice attracted by the warmth of the huge ovens and the numerous titbits that fell to the floor. Being infested with mice is a challenge for anyone, but as a teenager I really hated having to stamp my feet before I stepped into a room to scare them. Then in bed at night I'd lie there listening to the sound of them scurrying around the lino.

But the mice were cute compared to the cockroaches that loved the yeast used for the bread. There was nothing worse than switching on the light at night only to see ugly black insects scuttling everywhere.

It was my job to get coal for the fire in my grandad's bedroom twice a day and as I descended into the cellar with a brass bucket via a trapdoor on the shop floor I would be almost paralysed with fear at the thought of all the cockroaches lurking in abundance in the cellar. As I shovelled the coal I'd catch glimpses of their crackly coats as they glistened amongst the coal and on the roof above my head.

So although the bakery business meant an improved standard of living for the family, it came at a price. Mum and Dad worked themselves to the bone and the stress of the business took its toll. This, combined with the fact they both smoked and took no exercise, resulted in them both becoming very ill before my teens were out. Yet even in times of enormous pressure and stress my sisters and I knew that we were loved more than anything.

Mum in particular was a great influence in my life and she certainly shaped my personality and character very positively. She taught all of us girls to care for others. When we lived in the bakery she used to note the customers who didn't have much money – generally the most elderly of the community – and help them out whenever she could. The customers would come to the shop and order hot lunches, usually things like meat pie and peas, but Mum would not take a penny from the poverty-stricken pensioners.

I remember one day taking a hot meal to an elderly gentleman close by, and quietly telling him Mum didn't want payment. He was confused. 'Why?' he asked me. I told him I wasn't sure, just that 'Mum said it was a gift'.

A big smile crept across his face as he put his money back in his pocket.

'Tell your mum this is the kindest thing,' he told me with a tear in his eye. I always felt happy when I was the bearer of Mum's good deeds. It taught me the real benefits of kindness and humility at a young and impressionable age. When I talked to Mum about it in later years she just insisted it was nothing and that we were the lucky ones to be in such a privileged position.

There were so many examples of these acts of kindness and generosity and Mum was certainly admired and loved by many in her life for sharing her possessions and her time at every opportunity.

It was during the 1970s, when my parents were on their way back from visiting my sister Susan, who was at that time living in Bermuda and working as a teacher, that the full impact of Mum's non-stop labouring came to light.

On the way home Mum, now in her mid-fifties, was very ill, complaining of severe chest pains. Although she recovered a little a few weeks after coming home, Mum soon had another attack of pain. I was in the house at the time, and I distinctly recall the noise Mum made when the pain came. She was obviously frightened and in shock, and we all were too.

Once we got her to hospital they diagnosed a large myocardial infarction (a heart attack) and she was admitted to the Intensive Care Unit.

The prospect that Mum could die was unfathomable and the whole family was devastated. We waited long days and nights for her to improve and recover. To everyone's utter relief she did. But it was clear now that Mum needed looking after and time to convalesce, so Eileen duly left college to help out.

It was hard to keep Mum stress-free but we rallied around – until disaster stuck again. Six weeks after Mum's scare, my father had a heart attack too and was himself admitted to hospital.

Suddenly my sisters and I had the double worry of trying to keep Mum calm and look after our father during his rehabilitation. On top of that decisions had to be made about the future of the bakery.

One evening I came home from college to a gathering of relatives. Mum and Aunty Pat wanted to talk to me. I was asked to leave college and abandon my A level course as my parents needed financial help. Aunty Pat had even spotted a job for me, a 'dispenser' post in Boots the Chemist.

I was devastated that I had to leave my studies. At the time I'd been doing my A levels at Paddock House Grammar School Sixth Form College and the short time I was there had a lasting effect on me. But I had to get over the disappointment quickly. My family needed support and there were too many other things to worry about.

Mum and Aunty Pat also talked to me about my future career.

'I think you'd make a really lovely nurse, Sheena,' Mum told me. 'Once you're eighteen you could start your training.'

The idea certainly appealed to me. Nursing was a popular vocation in our family. When I was young Mum had been a health care assistant at a nearby institution for the mentally ill called Calderstones, my Aunty Pat had trained as a nurse and my sister Anne and some of my cousins had also gone into the profession.

Mum talked with such passion about the people she worked with. She often recounted how sad it was that some 'inmates' had been admitted as children for shoplifting or other petty crimes and had spent almost their entire lives at Calderstones. She made a huge effort to try and help such patients as much as she could.

I also had done some work experience at Calderstones and loved spending time with the patients.

As Mum and Aunty Pat talked about my different options, the suggestion came up that I could even go on to train as a midwife. I decided that it was definitely something to think about. I'd spent a lot of time with Aunty Pat and her midwife friend Marion, who always had lovely stories about delivering babies.

'It's such a wonderful moment when mothers see their babies for the first time, Sheena,' Marion had told me. 'It really is magical.'

A job in a caring profession really appealed to me. The whole ethos of our family had always been about caring for others. Mum cared for us and there were big sisters who cared for the younger ones. When Anne came home Mum would always want to hear about what had been happening on the ward. She was so proud of Anne and held nurses in such high esteem.

'We'll all help you,' Mum said, with an excited look on her face. 'You have all these nurses in the family.'

Although I knew I'd be scared of the clinical procedures I felt it was the right decision. It was important for me to make Mum proud but being able to look after others was also something that appealed to my nature. So with plans to apply for my nurse training once my eighteenth birthday approached, I settled into my new job at Boots.

My working day was from 9 a.m. until 5 p.m. and every evening I would walk home to our 'new' home on Lime Street in Great Harwood, where we'd moved after selling the business.

One night I arrived home to find Mrs Cooke, my mum's old school pal, in our living room.

'Sheena, Mrs Cooke wants to ask you a favour,' Mum said. 'It's about Freda, her daughter.'

I knew Freda and her mum and dad from church as she used to sit in front of Eileen and me and we often used to admire her hairstyle. Freda also went to Paddock House where I had started to do A levels, although I never talked to her.

Mrs Cooke explained to me that she was worried about Freda.

'She never goes out,' she told me, 'so I wondered if you would invite her out with you.' I agreed to help, but when she'd gone I was a little reluctant.

Mum, however, wouldn't take no for an answer and said I had to go to her house that week and speak to her and that was that.

When I set off walking to Freda's I was in a stew. What would I say to her? I arrived outside the door and knocked nervously.

The door was opened by Mrs Cooke, who was delighted to see me. She invited me in and I was shown into the parlour, where I sat and waited until Freda came downstairs from her bedroom.

She was clearly as nervous as I was but we chatted about everything we could think of and it was all very pleasant. We had totally different backgrounds – Freda was an only child and had had a quiet life compared to mine – but the foundations of a solid friendship were formed.

Our friendship grew and after that Freda loved coming to mine and we had many happy times. Even when Freda went to college to train to be a teacher we still wrote and met up regularly.

Then tragedy struck. When Freda was in her first year of college her mum died suddenly. It was an enormous blow for Freda and her father. To lose your mum at such a young age was bad enough, but she had no brothers and sisters to share her grief. Luckily my family was able to step in and help in whatever way we could.

To this day Freda is one of my best friends. We have gone through so much together. I sometimes wonder whether Freda's mother somehow knew she was going to die young and made sure she had me and my family around her.

*

As my eighteenth birthday drew nearer I went for my nursing interview at Blackburn Royal Infirmary. It took place at the newly built School of Nursing on the grounds of the old hospital and I was taken to an office for what would turn out to be quite a formal interview.

It was conducted by the head of the school, a tall, fair-haired man called Mr Winterbottom. I was exceedingly nervous.

'Why do you want to be a nurse, Miss Murray?' he asked me.

'Um,' I began, feeling my face flush as he waited for my answer. I had anticipated this question and rehearsed the answer over and over, yet now I was dumbstruck. Finally finding my voice, albeit quite a shaky one, I told him about the work experience I'd done at Calderstones Hospital, and how much I'd enjoyed it and explained my pleasure in helping others.

I also spoke about my grandfather dying and how I had supported him in his later life and of course about Mum and Dad and their heart problems. I explained that my parents' sudden illnesses had had a massive impact on our family life, so I believed I would have empathy for other individuals in the same position.

My experiences in hospital as a child came into it too, although I don't remember mentioning individual nurses. The rest of the interview seemed to go well and I left feeling slightly overawed but pleased that I'd given it my best shot.

Then four weeks later a letter arrived emblazoned with the crest of the Blackburn and District School of Nursing.

I'd got the job and would be starting my training in a matter of weeks. I was overjoyed. The planning with Mum started immediately. I scribbled 'scissors, a fob watch and pens' on my list of things to buy. It was all so exciting!

Chapter 2

Staring at my reflection in the mirror I smoothed my hands down my plain turquoise dress. I could hardly believe the sight looking back at me. There I was in my uniform, complete with a white starched collar, apron, little cap and a fob watch pinned neatly on my frock. I was a nurse!

That morning I'd awoken with a huge knot in my stomach and a slight feeling of nausea. It was January 1974 and I was about to begin my first day of nursing training at Blackburn Royal Infirmary. The apprehension was overwhelming.

As it was my first day Dad had spared me the bus, kindly driving me the six-mile journey to the hospital from our home in Great Harwood. He chatted to me all the way but I could hardly speak for the nerves.

Arriving at the school building I took my place next to seven other nervous-looking student nurses, as we were met by a senior tutor called Miss Frankland.

Miss Frankland was pleasant and serious at the same time, and had what I thought was quite a 'posh' accent. She gave us our timetable and described the practical placements in the wards and departments and how we would learn the basics of nursing care.

The other students seemed friendly and were mainly local eighteen-year-olds like me, apart from one slightly older male nurse and a woman who was in her twenties and already a mother.

Some of the girls revealed they had been cadet nurses – a position for sixteen-year-olds who wanted to become nurses – so had the advantage of already knowing the NHS culture and systems. During the first few weeks there would be many scurrilous stories told during our breaks – some good and some bad!

Collecting our uniforms had created a great flurry of excitement as we were led in an orderly procession to pick up the various items that would complete our look. Measurements had been taken earlier and we couldn't wait to see our new garb on.

Once I reached the front of the queue I was handed a brown box with my name on it and a leather belt tied round the middle. Dirty uniforms were to be placed back in the box to be laundered and starched on a weekly basis, I was informed.

Opening the box I lifted out the turquoise dress that would from then on identify me as a student nurse. It was a plain A-line frock with a zip at the front and it came with eight stiff white detachable collars. Attaching a collar to the dress proved to be quite a struggle but the ex-cadets quickly showed me and the other new girls the ropes. Likewise the aprons (of which we had seven) and the caps (a rotation of three), had buttons which were embedded in starchy material and difficult to free with your fingers. Eventually though, with a little help, we were all dressed and standing there proud as punch, giggling and admiring our new looks. When I looked at my reflection in the mirror it filled me with such emotion that I almost cried!

I would soon learn that it was essential to have our uniforms just so. Woe betide the young nurse spied with so much as a button out of place. She would undoubtedly face the wrath of Sister Schuster, a senior member of staff in charge of Ward Six, who would bellow across the ward. Never mind if a patient needed a bedpan, off you'd run to get the button replaced.

When I look at old photos of me now from those early days I do think the uniforms were lovely. The original nurses' attire was derived from the nuns' habit, which led to the name 'sister'. It was designed to help identify the carers and to promote adequate hygiene.

There is no doubt that to this day a uniform worn well can promote a feeling of safety and give confidence to patients receiving care, but I am not sure the same applies to maternity. Later in my career I helped to spearhead a shift away from similar uniforms for midwives, as I believed it was unnecessary. In maternity care the 'patients' are generally healthy women who are about to make a life transition to become a parent. Building a relationship with a woman and her family based on a partnership rather than one where the health professional is 'in charge' seems preferable, and therefore the clear distinctions of strict uniform are not necessary.

*

So back in 1974, with our transformations complete, Miss Frankland took us on a tour of the wards. I was immediately aware of the hospital smell (clinical scents mixed with mustiness) as I soaked up the environment, the patients, the staff and the bustling activity.

'This is my life now,' I thought excitedly, as I watched the medical teams working all around me, caring confidently for their patients. 'I'm going to work here!'

As I crossed the wards wearing my smart uniform and beaming from ear to ear, I noticed patients and relatives were already acknowledging me and smiling back. They didn't know I was a novice, finding my feet on my very first day. Instead the uniform gave them assurance about my prowess as a nurse. Was I up to the challenge? Well, I was going to give it a good try, and felt enthused at the prospect.

And so my baptism of fire began. The first ward I worked on was Ward Two, which was in a new section of the old Blackburn Royal Infirmary hospital. I may have looked the part but I was still very young and naïve and would quickly learn that I was in need of a thick skin and a strong stomach.

I had come from a family of girls, with a mother of firm moral standing, so it was more than a shock to observe some of the more intimate nursing and medical procedures for the first time. For example, it was only as I was allocated to the male side of the ward that the reality dawned on me that I'd be expected to give men bed baths.

Beforehand, my little group of student nurses had been shown how to carry out the procedure in one of the classrooms, with one of our peers lying fully clothed on a bed.

'Make sure the patient is warm and comfortable and not exposed,' our teacher had instructed. As we watched and learned, jotting down observations in the little notebooks we kept in the pocket of our uniforms, it had all seemed fine – but now I'd have to do it for real.

It was just days into my stint on Ward Two that I was first asked to accompany a senior nurse as she washed a male patient who was really quite unwell. My stomach churned as she instructed me to stand on one side of the bed while she took the other.

'I'll wash and you can dry,' she said.

After wringing out a flannel that had been soaked in warm water, the nurse gently washed the man's face, arms and chest. I followed suit, drying with a soft towel. Knowing what was coming next I took a sharp intake of breath.

'Shall we wash down there or hold the sheet up, while you do it?' the nurse asked the patient. The poor man was very ill but clearly bashful.

'I'll do it,' he mumbled. I was so relieved. Of course the time did come when I was forced to overcome my embarrassment and carry out the task by myself. Being very shy I never wanted to look but I knew that I had to be professional and get over that feeling. The last thing I wanted was to make the patients feel uncomfortable, so I'd do my best to get on with the job then save my blushes for the moment I walked away. To be honest the bed baths turned out to be tame in comparison to the pubic shave I later had to give one man.

I really loved caring for people but those first few months of learning how to carry out and cope with the clinical procedures were a massive learning curve for me. The parts of my training where my duties included helping with patient transfers, preparing instruments for operations and making sure the cupboards were stocked up and cleaned were all fine but students were also constantly invited to observe procedures or events that were seen as learning opportunities. I always knew I was squeamish, but during this part of my training my senses were to be tested beyond their limits.

Dealing with bodily fluids of every sort was routine, but when this was associated with trauma of any degree, I reeled. The first time I saw a blood sample obtained, I felt sick and had to force myself to look.

Keeping up my poker face as I carried out tricky or unpleasant procedures took a lot of work and to my horror I even found myself retching at times.

This happened for the first time as I helped pass a tube up a patient's nose. As I'd been taught, I instructed him to swallow when it reached the back of his throat. Every time the man tried to swallow he was nearly sick and as he gagged, I did too, having to turn my head away with embarrassment.

From then on in I had the same problem whenever people were being sick – or worse. If they were retching in front of me, I couldn't help gagging too. I'd swallow hard and avoid breathing through my nose but it was like a reflex reaction and I'd feel the saliva building in the back of my throat.

Seeing a patient crying also affected me. As Mum always told me, 'Your bladder is behind your eyes, my girl,' and no matter how much I bit my lip, seeing patients distressed set me off too.

'Sheena! You should not be so sensitive,' my superiors told me time and again when they caught me comforting a patient, my own cheeks wet from tears. 'You've got to be the strong one.'

One of the saddest procedures to come to terms with was laying out a body after a patient had passed away.

The thought of just seeing a dead body for the first time filled me with absolute dread, let alone doing all the tasks that were required like tying the big toes together and washing the body. It's horrendously sad to think you are dealing with someone who is not alive any more.

When the time came for me to lay out the body of an elderly gentleman, I was joined by a kindly third-year student called Marion Walsh, who did her best to make me feel at ease.

'If you talk to the body as if it's alive it makes it easier,' she advised.

To demonstrate she gently stroked the man's hair. 'We're going to look after you, don't you worry,' she told him, speaking softly. 'You're OK.'

So from then on I did the same and it helped me to get over it. I used to wash faces with tears in my eyes but all the while talking to the patient and caring for them.

Marion was to become an important role model for me. Her approach was perfect and she was friendly and supportive and wonderfully empathetic with patients and their relatives.

She really took me under her wing and I admired and

respected her. Marion and I became good friends and went on to attend each other's weddings. Thanks Marion. You taught me so much.

Each ward at the hospital had strict routines when it came to cleanliness and I would spend a large amount of my training cleaning. In the morning we'd help the cleaners, the cadet and auxiliary nurses to go round and make sure that everything was spick and span.

It wasn't a case of looking to see what needed doing, as you would routinely scrub things that looked clean. The domestics would damp-dust the surfaces of the ward three times a day and we'd polish the sterilised, silver bedpans until they gleamed.

You had to make the beds in a certain way. We didn't have duvets, just blankets and sheets. When we made the beds we did 'hospital corners' where the sheet was neatly folded and tucked under the mattress. All the corners had to go the same way with all the beds neatly aligned. However, while the wards looked neat and precise and patients had lovely clean beds, they weren't always as comfortable as they should have been. Unfortunately the sheets were very tight and starched, which could cause pressure sores on bottoms and heels.

Every day I threw myself into my chores with gusto. From the word go you learned how to work hard and if you were viewed as a good worker everyone liked you. I'd always try to do my tasks as quickly as possible so that the sister would think I was a grafter.

These days the strictness and fierceness of the ward sister

has diminished and maybe the cleaning routines aren't as rigid. Now hospitals have contract cleaners, which I'm not sure is the best way of doing it. The cleaners move around and don't take ownership for the cleanliness of a ward. If they did, perhaps things would be different?

Having said that, a lot of the problems hospitals face today are down to the fact that so many bugs have evolved to become more dangerous as they've grown resistant to antibiotics. I believe MRSA would have come anyway whether nurses routinely scrubbed every inch of their wards or not.

If I wasn't speedily cleaning, I would be doing the beds, temps (taking temperatures) and observations. If this duty was undertaken in pairs we were taught never to talk over a patient or to hold a conversation excluding them. This was a job I really relished as it gave me a chance to chat to the patients. It was the thing I loved most about working as a student nurse. Being with patients, helping them to feel more comfortable and assisting them on their road to a speedy recovery was incredibly rewarding.

I enjoyed getting to know them all and making them feel as secure and happy as possible. While I sometimes struggled with the medical procedures, this was the side of nursing I most cherished.

Whenever we cared for a patient or gave them their medication we would record it in a Kardex filing system so that the next nurse would have all the details of their progress.

During my time on Ward Two there were lighthearted moments and on one occasion a Kardex was even filled in for a blackbird that had nested and begun to lay her eggs on one of the ward window ledges. One of the patients had spotted the nest and, as there had been a buzz of interest from everyone in the ward, we started to make daily progress reports for Mrs Blackbird.

The admission note read: 'Via sky with abdominal pains. No previous hospitalisation. No known allergies. Laid first egg at 11.10 a.m. Mother and egg doing well.' Then with every shift change we'd do a further Kardex report. It was lovely as it brought fun and laughter to each handover. To our amusement the national press heard about it and came to report on our little feathered friend. I was volunteered to have my photo taken looking through the window at Mrs Blackbird, which duly featured in the next edition of the paper alongside the story.

As my training continued I got to know all the tutors and one of my favourites was a lady called Mrs Waddicor. While she could be stern and direct in her manner, she definitely appeared to have a soft spot for me. I couldn't exactly describe our relationship as one of friendship, but she helped, supported and encouraged me and I'll always be grateful for that.

I remember being dreadfully nervous before one of my clinical examinations and when Mrs Waddicor saw the state I was in she took me aside for a little word.

'Just be yourself,' she told me. 'You can do it. We hear good reports about you all the time.' Her kind words gave me confidence and I felt instantly better.

For a trainee like me to get this amount of support was

quite unusual in those days when the 'norm' was for senior staff to be quite intimidating and authoritative. As a student new to the NHS, you soon learned to be appropriately submissive, to comply, and most of all to be respectful to those in authority. The hierarchies that exist to this day in the NHS are quite remarkable and as a novice witnessing this culture for the first time it could be frightening and confusing to say the least. So Mrs Waddicor's attitude towards me was unique and much appreciated.

Much of the terminology in NHS hospitals (and which continues to be used in the present day) is based on the armed forces, with nursing 'ranks' and 'frontline' workers, for example. I always found the regimented hierarchical structure interesting.

When I began my career in the NHS, the days of the matron were long gone but their legacy was still apparent. Matrons had once been the most senior nursing rank but in the late sixties they were replaced by 'nursing officers' following recommendations in the Salmon Report that the status of senior nurses within hospitals should be raised. Nursing officers were less clinical than the matron and the intention was that they would have a greater influence on organisational decisions.

I'd met one of the nursing officers during my first tour of the hospital. Her name was Miss Adams, and her 'rank' was instantly recognisable by the blue dress she wore with a frilly collar. She looked very smart and her presence inspired awe in the whole student nurse group. When she addressed me in person I could actually feel my knees shaking.

The next nursing position after the nursing officer was

the senior sister, then the junior sister. All the nurses' uniforms were the same style, with starched aprons and caps, so the colour alone distinguished the rank. Sisters wore navy blue dresses and frilly caps. 'Sister' was in charge of the ward or department and her position of authority was a given. Woe betide the petulant young nurse who dared to answer back! Such insolence would result in a very public dressing down or the nurse in question would be marched to the office for a severe scolding.

Many of the sisters I came across were fearsome. With autocratic leadership styles they ruled their wards with rods of iron. Funnily enough the male nurses promoted to 'sister' positions, and named charge nurses, were in my experience much less frightening.

Although still strict and obviously 'in charge', some of the sisters were more approachable and had the skill to lead their teams with gentler methods. Being naturally timid I always felt more at ease to do my job well on these wards.

The next nursing rank was staff nurse – a position either achieved by completing a three-year programme to be a State Registered Nurse (SRN) or training for two years to be a State Enrolled Nurse (SEN).

The difference between the two was that the SEN needed fewer qualifications to enroll on the course, but once qualified would spend more time at the bedside rather than organising the ward.

Student nurses were next in the pecking order, then the auxiliary nurses, who were non-qualified assistant nurses – like my mother had been when I was young. Lastly, cadet nurses were sixteen- to eighteen-year-old girls doing a pre-nursing course.

So each group knew their place and was usually fearful of the next rank up, who acted with according superiority. At meal times or break times the sister and staff nurse would go together and the junior staff would have theirs separately. As a rule, junior and senior staff never mixed except on the ward or area of work during a shift.

Just occasionally, due to the skill mix on the ward, there would be a time when it was necessary for me as a junior student nurse to go for a tea break with the sister. This always created a strained atmosphere and as I sat awkwardly stirring my tea I was largely ignored.

I remember the senior staff who started to break the mould. They tried hard to bring staff members together, whilst still maintaining respectful relationships. They were the ones I watched closely and from afar, as I wanted to emulate their style. One senior nurse, Sister Blenkinsop, was like this. She was very proficient and knowledgeable but also considerate and understanding of the vulnerabilities of students. She always used to smile and tried to put me at ease by asking how I was and if I had any worries.

But it wasn't just the staff who had to conform to the hierarchies. While I witnessed some extremely positive aspects of the system in the 1970s, there was definitely a belief that patients had to comply too, to do as they were told and to be good. And it was never more important for patients to behave themselves than when one of the ward's resident consultants did his ward round.

The consultants were the top dogs, the nearest things to

God, and each sister knew she should ensure 'her' consultants got everything they needed and wanted on the ward round, whatever it took.

Unless we had been chosen to be one of a parade trailing behind the consultant on the ward round, we student nurses were expected to disappear out of sight. Admittedly that was the preferred option as joining the consultant's entourage was petrifying. Whenever my turn on the ward round occurred I'd stand at the back with the junior doctors doing my best to hide in case – horror of horrors – I was asked something.

My anxiety at a consultant's imminent arrival would also extend to the patients who I knew were feeling equally intimidated as this grand man approached their bed. Almost always, after the doctors had done a round, patients would ask me to find out what the doctor had said. So whenever I could I would suggest beforehand that they think about any questions they'd like their doctor to answer. But even with my encouragement, fear often stood in the way of their ability to speak up at the crucial moment.

No doubt the hullabaloo on the wards before a consultant's arrival did little to ease their apprehension. As soon as we'd get word a consultant was on his way it would be all hands on deck, with beds being straightened and lockers quickly tidied. If the consultant arrived early during drinks time, cups of tea and glasses of water would be swiftly snatched from the patients.

Just occasionally all hell would break loose when a consultant arrived at the entrance of the ward doors, completely unscheduled.

This was definitely the case when I spied Mr Green, the god of surgery, walking towards me one morning. Tall and lean with short, fair, curly hair and small beady eyes, he was trailing a stream of young, white-coated doctors in his wake. Sister was nowhere to be seen and my knees almost buckled.

'Good morning,' I stammered. 'Shall I find Sister for you?'

Mr Green glared at me, clearly disgusted by our perceived disorganisation and no doubt my insolence at speaking to him directly. Then to my horror he turned on his heels (he had a slight limp) and walked off the ward without saying a word. When Sister came out of a room moments later to learn what had happened she was angry. 'Where has he gone?' she asked me.

'I don't know,' I answered, biting my lip nervously.

'What on earth did you say to him?' she barked. Without waiting for me to answer, she brushed past me, red-faced, and went in pursuit of the master. I immediately made myself scarce.

Although during my nursing training I grew accustomed to the pompous air of many of the consultants, one incident deeply upset me. It happened in my final year when one of the hospital handymen was on our busy ward doing maintenance work on the bedside lockers. I was very fond of this particular man, whose name was John, as he was Irish and reminded me of my dad. He was a softly spoken man, but friendly, and he always had time to talk to patients as he went about his work.

The regime of this particular ward was such that the

consultant would come at 10 a.m. each day to see patients who had had surgery the day before. But on this occasion he arrived unexpectedly at 9 a.m. and bustled in to find Sister.

The majority of staff saw him entering the ward and made a quick exit to get out the way. But John hadn't seen him and in our hurry to disappear we forgot to remind him to make a sharp exit too.

I was just behind a screen at the end of the ward when I heard a thunderous cry from the consultant.

'GET OFF MY WARD IMMEDIATELY!' he bellowed, making everyone jump.

As I peered, horrified, through the screen I realised he was shouting at John, who had stopped his work and was walking quietly and humbly off the ward, with his head down. The patients all looked appalled and tears prickled in the back of my eyes as I took in what I had just witnessed. John, a man in his late forties, being totally humiliated – how could that be right? I felt so bad for him.

While that memory still riles me there were also some funny moments where the consultants were concerned.

I can remember one patient, a sweet-natured lady called Jessie, who with her few teeth, smoke-damaged complexion, thinning hair and mottled skin on her legs, looked much older than her years. Jessie had spent many years working as a prostitute and had sadly contracted syphilis. The disease had gone untreated and had affected her brain and she was in hospital for some investigations.

She was being treated by the senior ward consultant, Mr Bold, a swarthy, short man who used to wear a showy gold stethoscope round his neck. As he arrived on this particular day I was invited to observe proceedings.

As we approached Jessie's bed we saw that she was blissfully busy enjoying a cigarette – despite the fact that Mr Bold had previously told her she must give up as it was bad for her health.

To the amazement and horror of the team present on the round – we should have noticed the cigarette and removed it – Jessie apologised, took a long lingering drag of her 'fag' then passed it to Mr Bold with a wink and the cheeky request: 'Can you dock it please, cock?'

Without a word Mr Bold did as he was told, and as I scanned the faces of the senior nurses and the other doctors, I could see they were trying hard not to laugh. I will always remember Jessie with fondness.

As part of my nurse training I had to do a placement for three months in a department that wasn't classed as general nursing. This could be a specialist area such as mental health (psychiatry), children's nursing or maternity (obstetrics). It was my choice and I immediately decided to opt for maternity.

As well as the stories from Aunty Pat and her friend Marion, I'd been inspired by the enthusiasm of two of my friends Una and Veronica, who were 'pupil midwives' as students training in midwifery were called back then. They often talked with passion about the wonder of birth and how they felt they were helping women positively.

The maternity unit was at Queens Park Hospital, an ugly old building that had once been a workhouse for the destitute. Many local people remembered tales of the workhouse and disliked the hospital because of that reason.

But for me being on the maternity unit was a lovely experience. I loved being with the mothers and enjoyed learning how to help them when their babies were born.

As on previous wards I was expected to carry out the basic nursing tasks of checking the women's blood pressures and temperatures, but I also learned new skills such as assisting and supporting mothers to breastfeed and bathe their babies. It was a lovely experience helping a new mum to support and gently wash her tot in a bath. It was wonderful to see the babies also responding to the pleasant temperature of the water, wriggling their tiny toes and fingers, and I found it fascinating to watch how the mothers responded to their babies' cues as their natural maternal instincts kicked in. I loved snuggling up to the babies too, if the mother didn't mind of course!

I continually made notes in the small student nurse notebook that I'd been told to record all my experiences in. There was even a section for 'observed births' but while this was exciting I knew that it was unlikely that I'd get to see a baby being born. There were already more than enough pupil midwives and junior doctors floating around who needed to witness a certain number of births before they could start to deliver babies themselves.

My last shift was on a Sunday and I was pleased to see that Sister Livesey was in charge that day. She was the most senior sister, aged about fifty-three with greying straight hair and glasses, and I liked working with her as she was strict but also gentle and pleasant. That morning, as I was helping to restock the cupboards and do the routine cleaning, she called me over.

'Murray,' she said, addressing me by my surname. 'Would you like to come into this room with me? This lady is about to deliver.'

She didn't have to ask me twice! Quickly I grabbed a mask out of the glass jar next to the labour room (all staff were required to wear them to cover their noses and mouths before entering the room) and followed Sister Livesey inside.

In the labour room Sister Livesey began to put on her rubber gloves and a cloth green gown like the ones worn in the operating theatre (these were folded up inside a sterilised pack that contained instruments to help at the birth).

Besides us the woman in her twenties was alone, as at this time husbands or partners weren't 'allowed' to be present at the birth. Instead they were instructed to either wait in a special room or stay at home until they got the call that the baby had been born.

The woman's labour was progressing quickly and after introducing myself I stood and watched, feeling a mix of excitement and nervousness that this was going to be the first time I'd witness a birth.

It was the woman's third baby and my first thought was that she must be in a lot of pain due to the noises she was making and her facial expressions. As it happened I'd arrived at the crucial moment and she was just starting to push.

'Do you want to help me?' Sister asked.

Stepping forward I watched as she got the delivery pack

ready. She instructed me to quickly open an extra gown and pair of gloves and drop them on to the prepared delivery trolley.

I was still unsure what Sister meant by helping, but I did what she instructed, as quickly as I could.

'Wash your hands,' she told me quietly, 'And hurry!'

The woman was really pushing, and I couldn't help being amazed at how calm Sister Livesey was.

'The baby is coming,' she explained. 'And if you put on the gown and gloves and put your hands under mine, I will deliver the baby, but you can see how it feels.'

I was amazed to be given this opportunity but quickly did just that. The mother-to-be was working hard and within minutes the baby's head started to emerge. Sister Livesey stood beside me and told me to keep my hands under hers. I stayed still as she gently supported the emerging baby's head, then watched, breathless, as the body slipped out easily with the next contraction.

'It's a boy!' Sister Livesey announced.

I watched in awe as the mother sat up and gazed at her newborn with a look of unparalleled delight. Quickly she gathered him up as he gave a gusty cry.

I was grinning from ear to ear too. It had been an amazing experience.

'Congratulations and well done!' I said to the proud mother, who was hot and sweaty and gazing into her baby's face with a look of pure love.

Next I watched in wonder as the placenta (afterbirth), deep red and meaty, was delivered. I was absolutely dumbstruck by what I had seen and participated in. It had all been so quick – was I dreaming? I fetched the phone so the new mum could call her husband and then once both mother and baby were settled and happy I went with Sister to check the placenta.

She demonstrated how this was done, carefully explaining the importance of making sure the placenta and membranes were complete, with no parts missing. Although I had been shown the technique before I felt more involved this time as I had been part of the birth.

To this day I can still remember the surprise and pleasure I felt assisting with this birth. Later I went back to see the mother once more as she recovered with her new son. Gleefully, I told her how thrilled I'd been to be part of her special occasion and how the birth of her baby had made me feel that I wanted to become a midwife. Hers would be the first of many babies who I would witness making their way into the world.

Chapter 3

Approaching the patient quietly, I felt my heart pounding in my chest. In the eerie darkness of the ward, the man's face was pale and lifeless.

'Oh God,' I thought. 'I've lost a patient.'

Creeping closer I looked to see if there was any rise and fall in the gentleman's chest to indicate he was breathing. Nothing. Could I see flickering under his closed eyes? Not sure. I moved closer and touched his hand. To my horror it was stone cold.

Fumbling with his wrist I tried to feel his pulse and hovered over him to see if I could hear him breathing, gearing myself up for resuscitation.

'WOAH!' the man suddenly shouted, waking abruptly. I nearly jumped on the bed I was so shocked. It seemed he was very much alive.

Apologising sheepishly, I helped him to settle down again, tucking him in and asking if he wanted some water.

'Eh luv, tha' wants to give over fussin',' the man declared as I pulled up the sheets. 'Tha' gave me quite a turn!'

I was to learn that this was a common occurrence for

many nurses: apparently there is a fine line between sleep and death.

Working nights proved to be the hardest, as I forced myself to stay awake for twelve hours flat when my body was crying out for sleep. But the plus side was the companionship I felt with my night colleagues and the fact I was able to spend more time with patients. I enjoyed settling the patients down at night, then turning the lights out, satisfied that everything was shipshape.

After lights out there was a lovely calmness to the ward and even though the patients slept for most of the time I liked the feeling of watching over them to make sure they were all OK.

During the day there would always be a staff nurse or a sister in charge of the shift, but at night it was just me and another student nurse running the ward without any trained staff. If there was a problem or an emergency you'd bleep the night sister who did sporadic 'rounds' during the course of the night. But generally you were left to your own devices.

Understandably to begin with I did feel a little alarmed that if there was an emergency I would be the most senior member of staff on duty. I used to creep round the ward at regular intervals to make sure the patients were safe and comfortable and check if they needed anything.

On one night shift I was working on a busy surgical ward when I noticed that the bottle draining fluid from one of my patient's wounds needed attention. This was normally a job the porters dealt with so I duly called the office, but with all the porters already busy and having seen the procedure done in theatre I decided to deal with it myself.

The drainage worked with a vacuum effect and was either inserted near or into an operation wound. Beforehand the porters would use a suction machine to build up the pressure inside the bottle, which would then help remove the bodily fluid from the area and assist healing.

My patient's bed only had a portable suction machine, so I went into one of the cubicles where the suction was piped through the wall. A gentleman was fast asleep – I seem to remember that he had a chest problem – so very quietly I attached the bottle and waited for the process to be complete. But for some reason it wasn't working. I couldn't understand it; when I checked the attachment it fitted perfectly. I peered at it in confusion.

Suddenly the glass in my hand shattered into a million pieces with a terrifying bang. As I jumped out my skin I watched with horror as the chest patient awoke with a terrible start and stared at me with wide, shocked eyes.

Suddenly I realised my mistake. I'd attached the tubing to the oxygen instead of the suction. Oh my goodness, this was dreadful! To my horror the whole ward was awake, and I knew I would have to report my silly mistake to the night sister.

Unsurprisingly, I found explaining myself to the sister very difficult, and equally unsurprisingly I was in a lot of trouble – but even harder was settling down all the patients who thought World War Three had begun!

After a night shift I'd wait at the bus stop opposite the hospital, tired and cold and dreading the long journey home to Great Harwood.

Although Blackburn was only approximately five miles from my house, I didn't drive and needed to catch two buses to get to the hospital. This was difficult with shift work as the buses weren't reliable or regular.

One morning as I huddled at the bus stop, a car stopped and the male driver asked me if I would like a lift. He was a friendly man in his late forties who said he had just dropped his student nurse daughter off.

'I'm happy to drive you home,' he said.

It seemed kosher as I had previously seen him dropping off and collecting his daughter on several occasions, but I hesitated as I knew he lived in Blackburn and it would be taking him out of his way. But when he insisted I accepted gratefully and stepped into the car.

However, as soon as we set off he started to take me in the opposite direction.

'Do you know the way to Great Harwood?' I asked, concerned.

'Yes,' he replied, continuing to drive in the wrong direction with his eyes firmly fixed on the road. My stomach immediately lurched with fear. Something was definitely not right here.

'Please,' I insisted, voice shaking. 'My mum will be waiting for me and will be worried if I don't get home soon.'

In reality I knew that Mum wouldn't be worried until much later as the bus journeys took a long time. I felt sick and any tiredness I'd felt before had ebbed away to be replaced by abject fear and adrenaline as I tried to work out what to do.

I kept trying to think that this man was the father of

one of my colleagues – but then he put his hand on my knee and told me not to worry, and I nearly vomited with terror.

'PLEASE take me home as quickly as you can,' I cried, tears pricking in my eyes.

Suddenly he stopped the car and after conducting an angry three-point turn he accelerated back up the road in the direction of my home.

'You can drop me in the town centre in Great Harwood,' I suggested. The last thing I wanted was for this sinister man to discover where I lived.

He eventually agreed and, pulling up, he turned to me with a slightly fearful look in his eyes.

'Please don't tell my daughter about this,' he said.

'Of course I won't!' I agreed, desperate to get away, then I jumped out the car and ran home as fast as I could.

Bursting through the door I called out to Mum. We sat down over a cup of tea and I blurted out my story, tears of relief streaming down my face that I'd escaped unharmed.

Mum, in her usual calm manner, reassured me that I'd done nothing wrong but that I should never accept a lift from a stranger again. We also agreed it would be best not to tell my colleague, as basically it would be her father's word against mine and I didn't want to make a bad name for myself.

I didn't sleep well that day and kept thinking how sad and frightening it was that one of my colleague's fathers would do something as unsavoury as that.

Thankfully, four months into my training I was spared the bus when I moved into the nurses' home at Queens

Park Hospital. But having only ever lived with my family this was still a huge step for me.

The nurses' home was a foreboding building erected in 1926 to accommodate the nurses who worked in the former workhouse. The establishment hadn't witnessed much modernisation since that time, apart from central heating and some basic toilet blocks, so it seemed old and dated.

However, my room was small and cosy with a single bed made up using hospital-issue linen and covers. There was a built-in wardrobe with a sink and a mirror and the toilet block was just down the corridor.

A matron called Mrs Darlton lived on the premises and was in charge of making sure all the young nurses weren't misbehaving. Mrs Darlton was a stocky woman in her fifties with glasses and greying hair that was dyed blonde. Cigarette smoking was one of her favourite pastimes and she would sit, puffing away, in an old office at the entrance to the home.

The word on the hospital corridors was that Mrs Darlton, while strict, wasn't quite 'with it', and because she enjoyed a drink or two you could sometimes get away with breaking the rules. Yet I wasn't so sure and decided I would do my best to stay on the good side of her.

I noticed that she often tried to befriend the resident nurses, always favouring those in senior positions. I suppose when I think of it now, Mrs D was rather like Miss Hannigan from *Annie*. Though she wasn't cruel to us it was always a struggle to get clean bed linen and basic provisions such as bread and butter.

When I arrived to 'live in', I was given the rules in no uncertain terms.

'Visitors must be out by 10 p.m.,' she stressed. Although this seemed strict my sister had lived in a nurses' home ten years earlier and recounted tales of how she wasn't allowed out at night at all without a pass.

At the time I'd recently rekindled my romance with my boyfriend Paul – we'd previously been an item at school, but had broken up when we were seventeen. Paul was working as a toolmaker in Blackburn and we were reunited thanks to one of the other student nurses who was friends with Frank, Paul's best friend. When she told me what Paul was up to I thought it would be nice to get in touch with him again so I called him and arranged to meet up.

We met at the bus station in Blackburn and the minute I saw him all my old feelings came flooding back. Paul's looks had changed from our younger years – he now had a neat beard, as was fashionable in the seventies – but his smiley eyes were just the same. I thought he looked very handsome.

We went for a long walk and caught up on the missing years. We also went for a drink and shared a kiss before the night was through. From then on we were courting again.

As our romance heated up, Paul would often come and see me for the evening and I am afraid to say his departure was often a good deal later than 10 p.m. However, I was not alone in my rebellion and it was pretty much the norm to spot other young men creeping along the corridors at night as they rushed to the bathroom then back to their girlfriends' rooms.

This being long before the days of mobile phones, there

was just one telephone in the corridor shared by twenty nurses. It was our only link to the outside world – and, most importantly, boyfriends – so tempers were often frayed if one girl appeared to be hogging the line to whisper sweet nothings to her beau.

Still, there was plenty of fun to be had and I soon settled in, forming firm friendships with many of the girls on my corridor. The camaraderie was amazing and we looked out for each other, knocked to wake each other up in the mornings and chatted endlessly in our friends' bedrooms following shifts. If one of us had a difficult or stressful day, we always had someone to call on. If I was feeling upset I would simply do a tour of the halls looking for the light under the doors of my special friends, which would indicate they were home.

One of my closest friends during my training was Sandra, a pretty and vivacious nurse with shiny dark hair and deep blue eyes. She was my next-door neighbour in the nurses' home and we were always sharing food, drinks and stories. I can remember Sandra patiently listening to my troubles on many occasions and she was always there for me.

Then there were my pupil midwife friends, Una and Veronica, who both hailed from Manchester and were a few years older than me. Una was small, dark and feisty and Veronica more placid, with fair hair. They talked a lot about their midwifery training and constantly encouraged me to consider the same career path once I'd finished my nurse training.

The two of them had wicked senses of humour and I loved their company. They were also great fun, and Paul and I frequently went on evenings out with them. Being older and from the city, they initiated us into the world of drinking games, Italian food and parties.

In fact we planned the party of all parties one summer in the staff sitting room. Food was organised (not a priority) and drinks bought. The music was provided by a record player in the corner. Friends were allowed to bring other friends and it was going to be a ball. Paul invited his friend Frank, and unbeknownst to me one of my friends had invited a girl called Lynne, who was an orthoptist working with the eye care team at the hospital. Very sweetly Frank fell for Lynne that night and went on to marry her, and since then they have been lifelong friends to us both.

When I entered my second year as a student nurse I faced my worst scenario when I was required to gain experience in the operating theatre.

Most of my friends had loved this part, and had relished the detail when we'd met up to compare notes about our different training placements. But with my squeamish disposition, being called in to theatre to observe operations was the stuff of nightmares for me.

I might have known what was coming but as much as I steeled myself, the first time I stepped foot inside an operating theatre was every bit as traumatic as I'd envisaged.

To start with I couldn't stand the smell, a strange aroma of anaesthetic gases and cleaning fluids. I didn't like the drama either and the fact that the patients were very anxious beforehand. But most of all it was the blood and tissues on display during an operation that almost made me faint.

I dreaded the moment I'd be beckoned nearer to the table to look at a damaged liver or a cancerous pancreas and if I'm truthful I regularly closed my eyes. I reasoned that I would never need to know how to remove an organ in my career so I wasn't going to look!

Another stomach-churning moment came for me when we were taken to Manchester University to visit the medical school. The purpose of the visit was to see the forensic department in action and to observe the work there.

It was all fine at first and I was chatting to a couple of the students in my group as we entered a corridor that led to the security door where we were to gain access to the lab. But the minute we were ushered through the door I was overcome by the distinct smell of formalin – a sweet but strong-smelling liquid used for preserving human tissue. I had smelt formalin previously when samples had been taken or tumours had been removed in theatre and so I immediately associated it with an experience I didn't like.

I certainly wasn't prepared for what I saw next. Huge glass cases stood in front and to the side of me which, to my horror, held body parts. The first one I saw was a man's head, dissected on one side to reveal his brain, and the internal sections of his mouth and nose. Ugh. I turned away quickly to find I was looking at a woman's pregnant uterus. The uterine wall had torn (a condition known as ruptured uterus) and a dead baby was protruding out of the tear. It was horrific but for some reason I couldn't avert my eyes. I started to feel dizzy.

'I think I am going to faint,' I told my tutor. 'Nonsense,'

came her sharp reply. 'This is a great way of learning about the human body, and will help your studies.'

Before I could say a thing my knees started to wobble.

'Please,' I said. 'I need some fresh air.'

So with a look of disgust my senior pointed to the exit where a doorman would let me out. He directed me to some steps outside at the back of the building where I immediately sat down with my head in my hands. It took me about half an hour to recover and another ten minutes before one of my group was sent to retrieve me. I was quite embarrassed, especially as not only had the others survived the encounter but a few seemed to be positively relishing the experience!

So did it make me a worse nurse, not being able to cope with such things? I don't think it made the slightest difference. I was still totally committed and simply decided I would focus on caring for the patients and leave the blood and gore to the doctors. And that's what I did, carrying on with my training and loving the interaction with the patients.

In fact, nursing gave me an invaluable insight into the ups and downs of life itself. To observe or deal with patients or relatives who had been given bad news was an enormous challenge. Dealing with the sadness of others who were older than me wasn't something I had been used to.

In the first year of my training I saw the heartbreaking reaction of parents as their critically ill son passed away and I did my best to comfort a mother and father whose child was terminally ill. For the first time it made me see that life can be cruel.

People reacted in different ways to grief and it was heartbreaking to watch. While some people cried immediately, others seemed trance-like and numb or even in denial.

I carefully watched how my seniors approached situations and I asked them questions. I once saw Marion dealing with relatives who had lost a family member and was moved by how full of compassion her face was. She always seemed able to say the right thing. It was as though she gave something of herself and I liked that.

When the time came for me to comfort the bereaved or those whose loved ones weren't going to make it, I tried to act intuitively, giving them space if they needed it or being there if they wanted answers or needed to share their grief.

One of the most heartbreaking moments was when a father whose young child had died sobbed on my shoulder, distraught with grief but at the same time thanking me over and over for helping.

As he cried, his pain so raw, I could feel the tears prickling in my eyes.

'It's OK,' I told him gently. 'Anything you need you let me know.'

At night these harrowing scenes would sometimes play on my mind and haunt me but I found comfort in knowing I was doing my best to be compassionate and kind to those whose worlds had been shattered so comprehensively.

During my three years of training we had to undertake four practical exams whilst being watched by clinical tutors. The exams were incredibly difficult to pass and there was always much discussion about them amongst senior students.

'When are you taking your part three?' would be a sentence heard regularly. All the students were nervous when preparing for their exams as the fail rate was fairly high. Hardest of all was the written exam that we had to sit at the end of our three years of training, which enabled us to pass the final stage before registration.

I remember being worked up into a complete frenzy before this exam, which would last all day. What would the questions be? Would I have enough time? Had I prepared enough?

I had worked hard for months and months leading up to this exam, revising and going through old papers. I so badly wanted to pass and as I entered the examination room it felt as though my heart would stop.

As I took my place at my desk and we were told to start I glanced round to see all my group, heads down and already lost in their work. Then taking a deep breath I started to write myself, wracking my brains for the right answers.

When we came out of the room there was a sense of relief until we made the mistake of discussing the questions and answers in the coffee room. As expected, paranoia set in when others revealed better, well-articulated answers.

The letter containing my exam result would be sent to my home address and for days afterwards I listened on tenterhooks as stories were told and retold about how 'lots of good nurses fail'.

'Remember Jenny?' one girl would announce, relishing the drama she was creating. 'She failed and was devastated.'

We knew the envelope revealing our results would be brown in colour and there was even speculation as to its thickness. 'If it's a bulky envelope, you've failed!' was a common myth.

The night before the results arrived I couldn't sleep. Mum and Dad had listened to me going over and over the scenario of failure all evening. In the morning Dad joined me in waiting for the letter to arrive before going to work, and we sat and drank copious amounts of tea together.

I kept going to the door to look for the postman, and coming back again empty-handed. When he finally arrived it was a surprise, and hearing the letters drop on to the floor with a clatter I dashed to the door.

There amongst the mail was my brown envelope. Oh no, it was thick! My hands were shaking.

'Just open it,' Mum said.

'I am!' I snapped back.

Pulling a letter out I scanned the page for the wording that would seal my fate. Finally I spied it there in black and white.

'I've passed!' I screamed, jumping up and down. I was completely elated, as were my parents.

Now a newly qualified nurse, it was time to consider my future once more. I'd never forgotten my three-month stint in obstetrics and the wonderful birth I'd witnessed. As well as hearing the inspiring stories told by Aunty Pat, Marion and my friends Una and Veronica, I'd now seen for myself how looking after women before, during and after their labours could be so rewarding. I loved working with new mums and their babies and relished the opportunity to make it my full-time vocation.

'I've decided to apply to be a pupil midwife,' I told Mum and Aunty Pat proudly.

After chatting to my sister Anne it was decided that I would benefit from doing the course at a different hospital. On Anne's advice I applied to Burnley General Hospital where she'd trained to be a nurse. Anne felt that the Edith Watson Maternity Unit, which was part of Burnley General Hospital, had a good name and that it would be near enough to our parents' home too. 'It's really progressive and modern at Burnley,' she explained.

So I duly put in my application and in a short space of time received a letter to attend for interview.

Arriving at the maternity unit at Burnley on the day of the interview I was impressed to see it was housed in a new building – only about ten years old – which felt very different from the sombre old workhouse building I was used to. The windows were large and there was lots more space than at the maternity unit in Blackburn. It felt welcoming and I immediately liked what I saw.

My interview was with the head of midwifery, Miss Rishworth, a slim, smart woman with grey, well-manicured hair. She was quite formal but seemed nice, giving me the impression that the service her team provided was of a high quality. Welcoming me to the maternity unit, she invited me to take a seat.

'Why do you want to be a midwife?' she began.

Although the obvious answer might appear to be that you like babies, my aunty had already warned me that was the last thing I should say.

'Make sure you talk about what a privilege it is to be

there at the beginning of a new life,' she told me. 'And talk with passion about how you want to help.'

So with Aunty Pat's advice ringing in my head I explained how midwifery and nursing ran in the family and how much I'd enjoyed my twelve-week maternity placement.

'Witnessing a birth and how the midwife can help was wonderful,' I told her.

Miss Rishworth nodded and smiled encouragingly. So far, so good.

'What really matters to you?' she asked next.

Gosh, I wasn't entirely sure about how to answer this at first and had to give my answer some thought.

'Um, my family matters the most to me, I suppose,' I eventually replied. 'And the relationships within my family.'

Again Miss Rishworth nodded and after a few further questions it seemed my interview was over. I left feeling happy with my answers but also hoping that I had said enough to convince her I should get the job.

It took about a month to find out whether I'd been successful or not but I was ecstatic when the letter arrived offering me a position as a pupil midwife at the Edith Watson Maternity Unit.

A few weeks later, in May 1977, Paul helped me to move my belongings into Bennett Johns House, a staff residence in the grounds of Burnley General Hospital.

Moving to the next town was a big deal for me and I felt very brave. It seems so naïve now when I think how young people, my children included, travel all around the world, but still back then I felt every bit the adventurer.

Blackburn and Burnley were both old cotton mill towns,

once booming and vibrant and now somewhat faded. But the similarities stopped there. Even though geographically the towns were close they were polar opposites as places of work. I was soon to learn a different Lancashire accent, different culture and meet a wonderfully friendly bunch of midwives who would shape my future.

On my first day I arrived at the maternity unit with about ten other pupil midwives, many of whom were living with me in Bennett Johns. There were three local girls like me but the others were from different parts of the world including Malaysia, the Seychelles and India. Meeting these international students was exciting for me, as, apart from French friends, I'd never really been in close contact with individuals from other countries.

Our training would be crammed into an intense twelve months, which was very full-on considering that these days State Registered Nurses have to do an eighteen-month course to become a midwife and the training is university-based.

The midwifery school was located up a flight of stairs from the maternity unit and there my contemporaries and I were warmly greeted by Miss Cawthra, a senior tutor within the school. I remember her vividly. She was small with glasses, very straight short hair cut into a bob, and a fringe that settled just above her eyebrows. Miss Cawthra had a lovely smile but, boy, was she strict. Yet her 'jolly hockey sticks' character endeared me to her and her palpable passion for midwifery was infectious.

'Good morning, gals!' she'd trill in her posh, cut-glass

accent. This was quite a novelty for Lancashire and we were all mesmerised. You couldn't not listen to her – firstly you'd be in trouble, but secondly she was just so interesting.

Miss Cawthra was also good friends with Marion, Aunty Pat's friend, having worked with her years before. I think this connection gave her and me a kind of bond, although she'd never have admitted to it. I always suspected she was being extra nice to me because she always seemed to make the time to speak to me, whether it was as I came into the room for a lesson or when I was leaving at the end of the day.

'What have you been up to, Miss Murray?' she'd ask. 'How is your aunty, Miss Murray?' 'Are you enjoying your work, Miss Murray?'

I really liked learning from Miss Cawthra and the skills she taught me were to come in useful throughout my career. Interestingly, years later, in 2003, I wrote an article that was published in a midwifery journal and received a letter from her saying how proud she was and how she'd never forgotten me. We wrote to each for a while but then on the last occasion she didn't reply so sadly I don't know what happened to her.

After meeting Miss Cawthra on that first day we were taken to collect our uniforms. And just like my first day as a nurse I felt immensely proud and thrilled when I tried mine on. It was so different to the one I was used to: a white dress with no starched collar and a white belt. The white belt was exchanged for a blue one in the second half of the year so that you were identified as a senior student. Importantly we were presented with a book in which we would log the details of all the births we witnessed and 'conducted' during our year's training.

As a group we were given a week's introduction to our course, and what was expected of us. When the time came for us to begin our clinical work, I was reminded of the giddy nervousness I had felt as a student nurse.

I found midwifery very different to nursing. While the fundamental caring element to the roles was the same, as a midwife there was more of a focus on assisting and facilitating rather than 'making better'. Most of the women weren't sick but healthy individuals moving through the most exciting time of their lives.

In the early days, and to a lesser degree throughout my training, I didn't have the same instant job satisfaction as with nursing, where I could make a difference within seconds to a sick person's wellbeing. As a student nurse I felt very valued and got a lot of joy from helping sick people to feel better. Of course some people couldn't get better but even in those cases I was able to make what time they had left more comfortable. Whether I helped them to get out of bed, took their stitches out or cleaned their wounds, I got lots of feedback. Sick patients were always really appreciative and grateful and I liked the feeling that I was helping to ease their pain.

I found it very different with pregnant women. These women weren't ill: they were in hospital to have a baby and I was there to help. Although many of the women I cared for were anxious and concerned about their baby's welfare at and following the birth, I was aware of a certain strength and self-confidence in pregnant women, which enabled them to support themselves. Women used to thank me, of course, but it wasn't said at the same level of intensity. Understandably they were too busy enjoying their baby and new life.

I was to learn that the job satisfaction in midwifery came from doing less *to* individuals and doing more *with* them.

Chapter 4

My legs began to wobble and my face felt hot and flushed as a familiar and dreaded feeling of clamminess crept up my chest.

Oh God, I was going to faint. Right in the middle of the crucial moments of a baby's birth.

Keen not to end up in a heap on the floor, I quickly apologised and dashed out the room into the cool corridor. Finding a chair I sat for half an hour with my head between my knees, feeling utterly dismayed.

Feeling faint was bad enough but feeling faint while witnessing my first birth as a pupil midwife? Not good, Sheena.

Earlier I'd been invited into the hot and stuffy labour room just as the labouring woman was beginning to push. She was laid flat on her back, with her legs pulled up and propped against the waists of two midwives (one on either side of the bed). The mum-to-be was clearly pushing with all her might but finding it a real struggle. As I observed I started to feel panicked. I was convinced that this baby would never come out.

As the baby's head finally became more visible, one of the midwives performed an episiotomy, where a pair of scissors is used to cut into the woman's perineum to create more space for the baby to emerge. I knew about this procedure but it was the first time I'd seen it. Although my instinct was to close my eyes I'd managed to keep one open knowing that at some point I would have to do this. It was not pleasant.

Suddenly I felt completely overwhelmed, not just because of the stifling heat but also due to the intense atmosphere in the room. Dizziness quickly set in.

As I sat despondently outside feeling like a great big failure, I was approached by one of the more senior midwives.

'Don't be put off,' she told me kindly. 'It's always difficult at first and it happens more than you'd think.'

When I recall the intensity I felt for that first difficult birth I can understand how some birth partners feel when they are suddenly brought into a situation where their loved one is in the final stages of labour. It's not necessarily so much what is happening physiologically to a woman's body, but more about how women are cared for during their labour.

When I'd walked into the labour ward the woman had appeared to be in a vulnerable position, flat on her back, trying to push upwards and against gravity. Episiotomies were performed routinely in those days on all women who were having their first baby and had been done to help speed things along. However, to my inexperienced eyes it had seemed really barbaric.

I was also witnessing the birth out of context. I hadn't met the mother previously or seen her as her labour was progressing. I didn't know her partner or the staff attending to her so it seemed all the more extreme.

It's for this very reason that I wonder what affect reality TV programmes about maternity care, such as *One Born Every Minute*, are having on society's view of childbirth. The viewer sees an edited section of a woman's labour and birth, often chosen for its dramatic content. It is completely different from being in a room with a woman for her whole labour and birth, especially if she has minimal or no unnecessary interference.

During the year I had to witness twenty births and deliver forty babies, which often meant I'd be hauled into a room just as a woman was about to give birth. However, I also got to see many births in context. As a result of those, I learned not to panic.

In fact I soon learned that 'conducting a delivery' was quite an organised and regimented process with a strict protocol for everything from opening sterilised delivery packs to when you should 'instruct' the mother to push.

Labouring women weren't allowed to eat or drink in labour in those days and were given medication to reduce acid in their stomach. This was done to prevent problems occurring if the woman needed a general anaesthetic, for example a Caesarean section. But women were often hungry and had bad breath due to ketones in their bodies. Nowadays practices have evolved and women are encouraged to eat if their labour is progressing normally as it helps to keep their energy levels up.

In the 1970s and 1980s there was much more focus on procedures and processes as opposed to caring for women as individuals. This was a very different attitude from that held today, now that women have so many choices with their birth plans.

When a pregnant woman rang up to say she was in labour we would ask her to come in for a check where she would be directed to an admission room. This was a small room where an initial examination would take place, checking that mum and baby were OK, and establishing whether labour had started or not.

I felt this admission process was almost like a disrobing exercise as we duly asked them to remove their clothes and put on a hospital gown or nightdress. They weren't 'allowed' to wear their own in case they got soiled.

With the woman now adorned in a (usually backless) gown she'd be asked to produce a urine sample. The check would be done systematically, in order, so that no part of the examination would be missed.

If the woman was in labour, she was given a full pubic shave, an enema and then a bath, whether she liked it or not. It wasn't as though these procedures were intentionally forced upon women, it was just that this was how it was done.

From my recollection, women rarely vocalised their dislike to these procedures but neither was there any process of informed consent. There was no information about the procedures given either. These days the advantages and disadvantages would undoubtedly be listed for women to decide if they'd like to go ahead or not.

There wasn't much information about pregnancy and birth either – especially compared to today where the internet is easily accessed and women are able to look into the interventions they are offered.

Admittedly there weren't as many choices, particularly in areas such as screening in pregnancy. In fact 'choice' was a word that was hardly used until the 1990s.

Instead just three things were written in the woman's notes: shave, enema and bath. In that order and to be ticked when completed.

I first observed this whole 'admission procedure' during my stint on the delivery suite.

It was uncomfortable to watch and when my turn came to carry out a full pubic shave – removing every strand of hair from the woman's genital area – I felt very embarrassed about what I had to do. Young people today may go to beauty salons and pay for similar waxing, but in the seventies and eighties this was completely alien.

After the shave came the enema. This consisted of the administration of two full pints of green soft soap into the woman's rectum (back passage). The soap came in jars and we had to dilute the concentrate with hot water. Next a long tube with a funnel on the end would be pushed into the woman's back passage and the soap poured in. It was a common thing to hear the older midwives instructing the younger ones who were about to administer an enema to 'give it high, hot and a hellavalot!'

Once the task had been completed it was clearly difficult for the woman to keep so much liquid in her rectum. But yet we encouraged her to stay on her side and not to rush to the toilet, as the liquid would simply come out without having time to work.

When I think back to those times it makes my eyes water. Women in labour were already in pain with their contractions and feeling heavy with a full-term baby, so having water and soap inserted into their bodies must have been extremely uncomfortable.

Of course during our lectures Miss Cawthra had all the explanations as to why these actions were carried out.

'It's to ensure cleanliness,' we were told. 'The enema is given to clear everything out before baby comes.'

There was always the debate that enemas 'helped labour to progress' or 'prevented soiling at delivery', which was generally true, and I am sure there are still many advocates who believe the benefits outweighed the trauma.

Thankfully, step three – the bath – was the best part and was usually very much savoured by the expectant mothers after the previous procedures.

Even though there was a general culture of 'do as I say' in maternity care, as there was in much general nursing at that time, I did come across individual midwives who used to try to influence practice by encouraging pre-procedure discussions with patients.

One such woman was Mrs Woods, a senior midwife who worked with the night team. She was well respected and strict but also had a lovely manner with patients.

'Right, I'm going to give you an enema,' she'd tell women with her distinctive lisp. 'Where else can you get two pints of the best at this time of night?'

It might not have felt like there was much 'choice' or

'discussion' for them but the gentle manner with which Mrs Woods addressed her patients definitely put them at ease.

Working on the antenatal ward was interesting and very busy. Often women were admitted if they had problems such as pre-eclampsia (a potentially dangerous pregnancy-related condition associated with raised blood pressure and other symptoms), uncontrolled diabetes or their baby wasn't growing adequately. I was trained by the experienced midwives to monitor a range of medical problems and my training as a nurse certainly helped in these situations.

When women were admitted with severe pre-eclampsia there was always the risk that they could develop eclampsia and have a fit, which could be fatal for mother and baby. In the seventies and eighties women were cared for in darkened rooms with towels or sheets tied round the door handles to prevent the doors banging, which could provoke a fit.

Times have changed, and the care and treatment for some of these problems is radically different from my pupil days. Today's treatment for the same condition involves the use of drugs that research evidence has shown to be effective.

Although the antenatal ward was busy I really found myself on a steep learning curve when I started my stint on the labour ward, or delivery suite as it was known.

I was to witness all kinds of births, including breeches where the baby's bottom comes out first and tricky deliveries where forceps had to be used.

I found the first forceps birth I saw quite traumatic.

The labouring mother, Mary, had been pushing hard for

more than two hours and was exhausted. Her baby was lying in a posterior position, which makes it more difficult for the baby to be born, and was becoming distressed.

In those early days of my career women were nearly always laid flat on the bed for their labour. We now know that this is the worst possible position to be in – as they were forced to try to defy gravity and push their baby upwards – but then it was very much the norm.

Mary was lying down and her legs were placed in stirrups. Seeing a woman having her legs prised apart and placed in straps attached to poles at the foot of the bed becomes an everyday sight to midwives and doctors working in maternity units, but my first experience of the procedure disturbed me somewhat.

As instruments were used to pull out the baby's head I felt my heart racing. It was a huge relief when Mary's baby finally arrived safe and well.

I was also glad I'd survived another birth without fainting – which to my relief never happened again.

As I continued in my new role and built up my skills I started to enjoy the thrill of midwifery. I loved being part of the beginning of new life and witnessing the sheer joy on a mother's face as her pain disappeared and she met her baby for the first time.

Time and time again I would stand in awe, watching a woman with her baby nuzzling into her neck or suckling at her breast, exhausted and sweating but elated and wide-eyed. Being a midwife was extremely rewarding, and I was learning so much.

*

Eventually, after observing birth after birth, the time came for me to learn how to deliver a baby for myself.

Gowning up, I felt a tingle of excitement as I took the lead in the delivery with Julie, a very special midwife and mentor, guiding me.

'Just listen to Jo as she has her baby,' she had told me beforehand, 'and think about what you have learned already.'

When the time came for the woman to push I could feel my knees were knocking under the delivery bed. But I had a great big smile on my face as I remembered Miss Cawthra in the midwifery school teaching us how the baby manoeuvres out to be born.

I also marvelled at the mother, Jo, in front of me, who was about to meet her baby and was trusting me to help her. As I encouraged and supported her to push her baby out I had a great feeling of excitement and apprehension too. I wanted to do everything right.

Julie guided me every step of the way. There was no criticism, just occasional feedback.

I watched in awe as the baby's head appeared quickly (it was Jo's second baby). Jo had been given pethidine to ease the pain and was also using gas and air. As she moaned loudly I did my best to help her as I'd seen colleagues do previously.

'It's all fine, Jo,' I told her. 'You are doing great and your baby is almost here!'

As the head appeared I waited for it to turn as I'd been taught and then I wiped the baby's eyes with cotton wool swabs. The baby's body was still in the vagina and following practice I felt for the baby's cord round his neck. It was there but loose, so again as taught, I slipped it carefully over his head.

With one more push, a wet, slippery and glistening baby boy slipped gently on to the bed between Jo's legs. She groaned with relief and then beamed from ear to ear as she sat forward to pick up her new son.

I congratulated her quietly and placed a clean white towel over the baby to keep him warm. Then I took a moment to marvel at the mother and infant falling in love.

'You were brilliant,' I told her. 'Amazing.'

Julie winked at me as if to say so far so good. Then she guided me through the delivery of the placenta.

In those days all mothers had an injection of syntometrine when the baby's body was emerging, to help the placenta to separate and be delivered. Julie had given Jo the jab, and now we had to put some gentle traction on the cord to ease the placenta out. I found this quite hard at first.

'You musn't pull,' we'd been taught in school and during our early days. 'The traction needs to be consistent and sustained, but no pulling!'

I found this confusing at first but gradually learned what degree of tension was needed for the procedure. When the placenta appeared I sighed with relief. I scooped it up and plopped it into the waiting kidney dish on my beautifully prepared trolley.

Next came the gentle and methodical swabbing, and the careful bathing of the tender labia that looked battered and bruised.

Julie guided me through checking to see if any stitches

were needed. Jo, meanwhile, seemed unfazed, as she was busy checking her baby's fingers and toes.

She did need a few stitches, which Julie carried out with careful precision as I took note. Then after Jo had called her husband who was at home with their other child, we made her comfortable, checked and weighed her new addition and encouraged the first feed.

Jo was tired but elated when her husband and little one arrived and we left them to get to know the new baby some more.

Later on, before Jo went to the postnatal ward, I went to thank her and told her that she was the very first birth I had attended as a pupil midwife.

'I am so proud,' I said. We hugged and I told her once more how amazing I thought she was.

Max, her son, will be thirty-three years old now. I wonder what he is doing?

That night I went home and phoned Paul to tell him. By now we were very much in love and I enjoyed sharing every moment of my emotive journey to becoming a midwife with him. Although obviously I spared him some of the more gory bits!

Working as a pupil midwife I found the hierarchical attitude of some of the midwives more intense than in nursing. The demarcation between grades of midwives was palpable and could be quite intimidating. Bullying the midwife who was a grade below was almost seen as a rite of passage. This didn't begin or end with the midwifery staff. The obstetricians, like the consultants in the general hospital, were the masters. Their behaviour or mood influenced the atmosphere on the wards, and there were some who were intimidating to say the least.

But while there was the odd member of staff who made life difficult for the others and some subtle bullying certainly went on, there was also a lot of brilliant camaraderie on the delivery suite at Burnley and some real characters.

As a young student I was in awe of many of the senior midwives. I have particularly fond memories of working with a nursing officer based on the delivery suite called Miss Fenton. Miss Fenton was very strict but had incredibly smiley eyes that twinkled when she laughed.

She would also slap us in a playful manner. My friend Eileen often joked that these were her 'love slaps', as she only seemed to do it when she liked you. It was more of a tap really, and I was never offended by it.

While I liked her I was admittedly a little scared of her, as she was still quite an austere character. When she barked your surname across the ward you'd immediately set off running.

So one day, at the end of my shift, when I heard the cry of, 'Murray, come here!' I instantly wondered what I'd done.

'Now, Murray,' she said, when she had my full attention. 'I can't get to work tomorrow morning. You live by me. Can you give me a lift?'

Well, what an honour! I was totally taken aback and flustered and immediately went home to clean my old green Hillman Avenger car.

The next morning I was up at the crack of dawn feeling slightly nervous and worked up. What worried me more than anything was that the reverse gear on my car was broken. We couldn't afford to get it fixed professionally and although Paul would always try to mend our cars himself we also couldn't afford new parts. Consequently I was making do and always had to park in a place where I could drive in and out easily.

'You'll be fine,' Paul had told me when I'd confided my fear over the phone that night. 'Just don't get into a situation where you have to reverse!'

So, nice and early that morning I arrived at Miss Fenton's home. She was ready and jumped in with a brisk, 'Good morning, Murray.'

Setting off I immediately felt under enormous pressure. Here I was, having to make small talk with my senior manager and concentrate on driving. I drove with more care and caution than I'd done taking my driving test and was very relieved to finally arrive at the hospital.

But just as I rounded the corner into the huge hospital gateway I was horrified to find a big wagon coming out. The vehicles met in the middle and there was no way for me to drive round.

My heart nearly stopped. 'Oh my God,' I thought. 'I will have to reverse!'

As I gasped in horror, wracking my brains for a solution, Miss Fenton looked at me questioningly.

'Are you not going to reverse, Murray?' she asked.

'I can't,' I muttered, wishing the ground would open up and swallow me.

'What do you mean you can't?' she barked. 'Have you not passed your test?'

'No, the car doesn't have a reverse,' I admitted, going redder by the second.

Miss Fenton, to my amazement, actually swore. The situation was getting worse by the minute.

Jumping out the car I ran over to talk to the man high up in his cab.

'What?' he said scathingly. 'No reverse? You shouldn't be driving it!' Out he climbed and strode moodily towards my car. Then, as I stood there cringing, he pushed the car backwards with Miss Fenton still in it!

Biting my lip and with a face now as red as a beetroot, I got back in and drove into the grounds. Well, Miss Fenton just sat there laughing her head off! I'd never heard her laugh like that and she literally guffawed all her way into the building. It appeared to have tickled her so much that she told the story to everyone. I was mortified but after that Miss Fenton clearly had a soft spot for me and I'd get more of the little slaps whenever she walked past.

In fact it was Miss Fenton who instructed me to do my first 'solo' delivery where I'd help a mother give birth all by myself. This was essential for me to pass my qualification but I'd been dreading doing it. It was a big weight on my shoulders to know it would be entirely down to me with no senior member of staff watching (although there would be one just outside the door should they be needed).

'Right, come on Murray, you've got to do this!' she told me. 'Go in there and deliver that baby, and don't ask for help unless you need it.'

'Oh, do I have to?' I can remember wincing, anxious

about the responsibility. I knew full well what the answer would be.

'Yes!' she barked, asserting her point with a quick 'love slap' to my arm.

When I arrived in the room I introduced myself to Louise, a young primigravida (first-time mother) who was quite frightened and in the first stages of labour. Her husband Terry was also there.

Jane, the midwife going off duty, gave me a handover of Louise's progress and bid us goodbye.

'I'll come and see you and your baby tomorrow, Louise,' she smiled.

As the door shut behind her I took a big breath. So here I was alone without an experienced midwife in the room.

I felt unexpectedly fine, as I knew the girls outside were rooting for me and would be there in a shot if I needed them. I just had to concentrate and keep my cool. I wanted to succeed in my first solo birth and I felt proud to be in this responsible position.

With Louise on the bed, Terry and I took it in turns to rub her back and legs when she wanted us to.

As the labour became more intense Louise was clearly struggling. When the time comes to push the labour pain becomes more intense and women frequently get the 'flight' urge, either to give up or get out. Louise was sweating and red-faced.

'I can't do it,' she said, her face crumbling. 'It's too hard!'

'Yes, you can,' I encouraged, and Terry and I worked hard to help her through.

During second stage I became concerned about the

baby's heart rate and immediately called a senior midwife and a doctor to check.

They confirmed it was OK to continue so I listened in more frequently from then on. The baby was fine.

Pushing continued to be hard for Louise. She sat upright and used every ounce of energy she had to move her baby down, gripping Terry's hand so hard that her knuckles were white.

'I can see the head,' I told her. Then I explained that I would soon be putting in the local anaesthetic prior to doing an episiotomy. I can't remember whether or not I felt one was necessary but I do know that I would've been in serious trouble if I hadn't done one.

I still found episiotomies hard to handle and I suppose that was one task that freaked me out. To actually pick up a pair of scissors and cut into a woman's flesh was a huge challenge.

This is one of those scenarios where the ritual of the procedure helps to take your mind off what you are doing. You are taught to do the procedure in a certain way. It has to be carried out when the perineum (the skin between the vagina and anus) is at its thinnest, which is when the baby's head is well down and ready to be born.

The area has to be cleaned and injected with local anaesthetic and then the scissors inserted in a certain way. Concentrating on doing it right almost blanks out what you are actually doing in reality. Although remembering the delicacy and invasiveness of the task is crucial as it can be distressing for the woman or her partner.

There is still an interesting debate as to which is best, an episiotomy or a natural tear, and there is plenty of evidence and expert opinion on the matter. Either way, learning the procedure was no easy feat and in my latter baby-catching days I would only do an episiotomy if it was absolutely necessary.

Louise didn't protest, so with her perineum anaesthetised it was time for me to pick up the scissors and carry out the deed. Was this really the right time? With no one to reassure me, I just had to trust my instinct.

I performed the task quickly and although Louise didn't feel it I saw Terry wince.

The baby's head emerged with the next push and Louise put her hand down to touch the slippery skin.

'Oh, my baby!' she cried.

When her baby girl was born two pushes later, Louise cried out in delight as the pain vanished instantly.

'Louise, we have a girl!' Terry cried out.

They hugged and cried together in a very moving moment. It took me a long time to stop myself becoming watery-eyed when couples cried and embraced as they met their child for the first time.

With Louise and her baby settled and happy, I couldn't wait to leave the room to tell Miss Fenton and the other midwives.

'I did it!' I announced with a huge grin and sweat glistening on my brow. My hair was all tussled and I felt drained, but I was over the moon. I was going to LOVE being a midwife.

When I got back to Bennett Johns after my shift, I immediately rang Paul and my mum to tell them my good news. They were as thrilled as I was, especially Mum who always felt so proud of our achievements.

As we pupil midwives grew in confidence and experience we would find ourselves very much in the thick of it. On the night shift the senior midwives would sit in the staff room with the door closed and, keen to impress, we would not disturb them unless it was absolutely necessary. Instead we would carry out all the care for the women, delivering their babies and cleaning the rooms.

As ultrasound scans hadn't been introduced yet there were occasionally surprises during the birth, such as undiagnosed breeches, where suddenly we realised that the baby's bottom was coming first. This still happens today, but it is much less common.

On one occasion I delivered a baby that was just being dried after emerging from between the mother's legs, when the mother became agitated once more.

'The pain is back,' she said. 'I need to push again.'

My colleague immediately took a look.

'There's another one in here!' she exclaimed.

The mother was slightly confused but obviously preoccupied with giving birth again. Meanwhile her partner was ashen as the news hit him that he'd soon be a father of two! This happened more frequently in the seventies and many midwives (and parents) have tales to tell of this scenario.

It would often get very busy and if a problem arose one of us would dash to the day room and knock anxiously on the door.

When the door opened you'd get a glimpse of the senior midwives sitting around chatting, smoking and painting their nails. They even had a freestanding hairdryer in there, like the ones in hairdressing salons, which they used to style each other's hair! I find it hard to believe now and when I talk to other midwives that worked as pupils with me during that time, we debate how barmy it was. Interestingly, as far as I'm aware, no one ever complained.

We worked hard and while it was stressful at times it was also very rewarding. There was one special member of senior staff called Sue Smith who used to bypass the staff room and stay with us, working alongside us and helping out. It was as if this senior midwife knew how hard we worked and wanted to be different to the rest. She was a great teacher and asked us questions as we were working together.

'What are the outcomes of posterior position?' she'd say and I'd have to wrack my brains quickly for an answer. What a great way of helping us to learn! Tragically, Sue died last year, too young. Her friendship and work is missed by so many in Burnley.

Of course as my experience of delivering babies continued and I saw first-hand all the joy and wonder that new life brings, I inevitably saw tragedy and sadness as well.

There was one young couple who I'd originally met in the antenatal clinic who seemed to have problems from the off. When the woman came in to the delivery suite her labour was progressing slowly and she needed some help from the medical team. Her contractions were speeded up with the use of a drug called syntocinon, which was given intravenously in a drip.

When I performed a vaginal examination just before she started to push I noticed that the baby's head was very soft, like a bottom. Suspecting a breech birth the doctors were alerted and on standby.

But as the woman began to push her baby out I was shocked to discover that it was being born head-first. But instead of having a normal head the skull appeared to be soft and collapsed in.

Even worse, when the baby emerged it was clear its facial features were badly distorted. Trying not to alarm the parents, I did my best to remain calm and composed. I quickly passed the baby to the waiting medical team who immediately whisked it off while we prepared ourselves to support the parents psychologically. Tragically, although the baby had been born alive, it died very shortly afterwards. The doctors explained that the baby had been born with anencephaly, a neural tube defect where a major part of the brain, skull and scalp is absent. This condition is very rare – thought to occur in about one out of 10,000 births – and I had previously only seen photographs in midwifery textbooks.

The poor parents, I felt so badly for them. All they could do was hug each other and cry. In a moment their lives had fallen apart. I didn't have any children at this stage in my career but their pain was heartbreaking and I tried very hard not to cry too.

'What did we do that made this happen?' they asked me, completely bewildered.

As they looked at me for answers I felt lost for words. What could I possibly say to make them feel better? All I could think to do was imagine Mum and how she coped with crisis in our family – calmly and kindly.

'You mustn't blame yourselves,' I told them, my voice shaking.

Although I gave them all the reassurance I could they were clearly going to be torturing themselves for a long time to come. Thankfully they were able to go on to receive counselling and plan future pregnancies.

I have since learned that when a baby is born with an abnormality or is stillborn, parents immediately ask themselves if it was their fault when 99.9 per cent of the time there is absolutely nothing that could have been done to change the situation. That night when I went home I felt deeply affected by what I'd seen.

Through the course of my midwife training I was to learn that life itself is complex and full of surprises and sometimes those surprises are very unfair.

Keen to help grieving parents or those whose children had birth defects as best I could, I carefully watched others more senior to me. I observed the way they carefully and sensitively broke news to a family that their baby wasn't perfect. It is not easy and never got easier.

Thankfully now because of sophisticated screening tests and ultrasound scanning the birth of an abnormally developed baby is a fairly rare occurrence. However, the dilemma continues in a different but no less distressing way. When parents are informed during pregnancy that their growing baby isn't perfect they have to make harrowing decisions about whether to terminate their pregnancy or not, and even when a decision is made, the trauma often continues.

Of course, dealing with the births themselves – whether the outcome was joyful or tragic – was only a part of my job. As well as my stint in antenatal and witnessing and delivering so many babies on the labour ward, I also needed to get the relevant experience in other departments and wards within the maternity unit. These included the special care baby unit (SCBU) and the postnatal ward. These experiences were invaluable and while I learned so much there was a very short time to take such a lot in.

I didn't like the special care baby unit very much as I missed caring for women. It was difficult as we students weren't allowed to care for the really sick babies but instead simply had to feed the bottle-fed babies all day.

This was a novelty at first as the babies were often very tiny and cute. But I preferred it when mothers came to feed their baby and I could help them and chat to them.

I did get attached to some of the babies that were in for a length of time. Some would be in for several weeks and we would watch them grow, even seeing them smile for the first time before they were discharged home.

The hardest part of the SCBU experience was the interventions on the tiny babies. I was invited to observe treatments on babies that were deemed interesting as part of my training. But if a small baby needed intubating (where a tube from its mouth would be attached to a machine to take over breathing) or required an intravenous drip I found it hard to watch and I wondered whether the baby could feel any pain. They seemed so tiny to be coping with such invasive procedures. I knew they were potentially life saving, but it didn't stop me feeling uneasy.

On the postnatal ward I became well versed in the procedures carried out once a woman has given birth.

After having her baby a new mum would be given a bed bath and a midwife or auxiliary nurse would transfer her to the postnatal ward with her baby.

In those days the postnatal ward was a wonderful place to be. There was a relaxed and nurturing feel to the care, with mothers encouraged to rest. The comforting smell of freshly buttered toast wafted through the ward as new mums were offered hot snacks and biscuits to get their strength up and tea in abundance.

Morning also brought more slices of hot toast and milky coffee for the mums and in the evening they were tucked into bed with cups of cocoa.

Women having their first baby would stay in for five days and subsequent babies for three. If the baby was born by Caesarean section then the mother and baby would be discharged between seven and ten days later. It's such a difference to the care today, where mothers may go home after six hours if all is normal and the average stay is only one or two days.

The daily checks and routine care were time-consuming and extensive. Women would stay in bed for a couple of days, so for the first twenty-four hours they were regularly washed in bed by the staff.

Learning how to support new mothers as they adapted to their role and helping them to care for their baby was a huge part of my daily work on the postnatal wards. It was rewarding to help in those early days when both mother and baby wore L-plates.

Helping mothers to breastfeed their baby could be difficult as the rule was that babies were fed every four hours and if they woke up in between their designated feeding times they would have to cry or were bottle-fed water or given a dummy. But we would still try and give them as much practical assistance as we could. I would sit and chat with mothers, showing them how to get their babies to latch on the breast, which can be far from straightforward, especially for a first-time mum.

Some women found feeding easy and had few issues, others needed extra support and then succeeded, while others would find it hard and always be on the verge of 'giving up'.

I would also help women as they got to grips with the many new tasks of motherhood such as bathing, changing nappies or comforting their baby when it cried.

Babies were removed at night and placed in the nursery so that the mother could sleep, although 'rooming in' was being introduced, which meant babies could be next to their mother's bed in a cot. During my career practice has evolved and mothers and babies thankfully now stay together. But in those days, each mum would be offered sleeping tablets and pain relief to settle down for the night. Then the babies would be lined up in the nursery, and fed four-hourly. No more, and no less.

It was quite difficult as there would nearly always be at least one baby crying, and although we would try to settle them, there were usually only two members of staff coping with up to fifteen babies.

It was also routine practice to give a baby a supplement

of formula milk if he/she didn't settle, with or without the mother's consent. With the knowledge generally available at the time we believed we were giving the best possible care, though of course this would never happen now or at least it shouldn't.

We also promoted 'controlled' breastfeeding, for example women were advised to start off two minutes each side (each breast) and to increase the time each day until the baby was 'allowed' to suckle twenty minutes at each breast. We now know that most of these methods are actually not advisable to the physiology of breastfeeding and probably contributed to many women resorting to bottlefeeding unnecessarily. But at the time it was seen as best.

Just like on the delivery ward there were harrowing moments and one of the saddest things I saw was a woman who was suffering from a condition called puerperal psychosis – a form of mental illness that can be so severe the person is totally debilitated. This is an extremely rare condition and is quite different from postnatal depression.

The woman, Mumtaz, was expecting triplets and had been in hospital for a while so I'd gotten to know her. Tragically, at the time of the birth, one of the babies died, and in addition to her extreme and understandable distress, we noticed an ever-increasing change in her behaviour.

Mumtaz began to accuse us of trying to kill her. It was clear she thought we were the enemy and the fear in her eyes was disturbing. At the height of her illness she was sweating in terror and became increasingly aggressive towards us.

Caring for her was incredibly difficult and quite

frightening. Her family were distraught, as this wasn't the person they loved dearly and they couldn't understand what was happening. They must also have been worried about the care of the surviving children, while at the same time juggling their own immense grief at losing one of the triplets.

Eventually Mumtaz was transferred to a mother and baby unit in a psychiatric hospital and made a full recovery. I met her several years later while shopping in town and she looked so happy and healthy. Her children were doing well, and her wider family too. We talked about the little girl she lost and had a quiet moment together.

Later in my career I had a very special interest in supporting pregnant women and new mothers with mental health problems as I felt it was an illness often overlooked and treatment was and still is under-resourced.

My social life continued to be as full as ever and working at Burnley I made good friends with many of my fellow pupil midwives. As well as sharing intimate moments as we supported each other through hard times, there were wild nights outs just like in Blackburn.

Also Paul and I were very much in love and during that year we decided to plan our wedding.

There was actually no romantic proposal but the pair of us had talked openly about the fact we'd like to tie the knot. In a very practical fashion we saved up to buy a house and decided on a date to get married. We paid for everything ourselves, as our parents weren't in any position to help us financially.

I did get the excitement of choosing my fancy engagement ring, though, and I chose a beautiful antique ring, from Mary Milnthorpe's jewellers in Settle, Ribblesdale. We celebrated our engagement with a small family meal. I felt very happy and grown up to have a 'fiancé'!

Paul used to come and see me at Bennett Johns House whenever he could, and on occasions he would stay the night. But the rules of the residence were just as strict as the nurses' home and overnight visitors were a definite no-no.

Although we didn't have a live-in matron, there was a Mrs Jones who coordinated the running of the facility and worked office hours, and a couple of cleaners who believed they were in charge of us.

Kate was one of the cleaners, a Scottish lady who was a real stickler for the rules. She started work at 6.30 a.m. each day and didn't miss a trick. There was no way we would get a visitor out in the morning without her seeing them.

Consequently Paul would leave via my bedroom window at 6 a.m., which wasn't an easy task. As I watched him hanging off my windowsill and manoeuvring himself haphazardly to the ground below, my heart would be in my mouth.

I'd then have to stifle my giggles as he ran – half-crouching to avoid being seen – across the hospital grounds to his car. It may not have been the most elegant way to leave, but as far as I was aware he did always manage to escape unnoticed.

Chapter 5

Stepping into the house I struggled not to let the shock show on my face.

There in front of me the floor was strewn with rubbish and junk – plates of old rotting food, dirty nappies, dog hairs, dog food and empty cans. I couldn't believe that a family was living there, let alone a newborn baby. The stench was unbelievable.

I'd been called to visit this home as part of my ongoing training as a pupil midwife. Now on my 'community' placement, I'd been assigned to a midwifery sister called Jean Quinn and once again commenced on a steep learning curve.

Sister Quinn was in her forties and always dressed smartly in a navy dress with a grey overcoat and matching hat. She was also straightforward, honest and knew her job inside out.

Our weekly tasks included visiting houses to check on mums and babies and running antenatal clinics in the community at GP surgeries.

Sister Quinn had a small Mini and we would zip around from house to house. She had a special leather nurses' bag (called a Gladstone) that reminded me of a Mary Poppins bag, as so much appeared out of it. Inside were weighing scales, swabs, cotton wool balls, a thermometer, small towel, a small tin of Ster-Zac powder (used for dusting the baby's umbilical cord to help prevent infections) and a cord clamp cutter.

We visited all kinds of different homes, from large luxurious detached houses in the country to small terraced homes in built-up areas.

As we journeyed from home to home, seeing all walks of life, sometimes I just couldn't hide my surprise. Some of the sights I saw during times spent working in Nelson and Colne, old Lancashire mill towns, I will never forget. I didn't think such poverty existed in developed countries, and certainly not in England, but I soon learned that my sheltered life had shielded me from so many realities.

I think Sister Quinn loved the fact that I was totally impressionable although she always did her best to warn me.

'There are some problems here, so we have to be careful,' Sister Quinn warned me en route to the home with the rubbish-littered floor. 'The house is very dirty and may not smell very nice, so pay attention to where you sit.'

I didn't know what to expect really, but was left speechless as we stepped in the door. Not only was there dirt and debris everywhere, but furniture was sparse and the whole house was damp and cold.

What surprised me the most was the apparent acceptance of the situation by the family. I soon realised this was normal to them and that I couldn't let the mother see my disbelief. I wanted to support her and didn't wish to make her feel awkward.

I remembered what Mum always used to tell me: 'You are better than no one and no one is better than you,' and I really started to think about what life must be like for families who lived in such conditions.

Another revelation was being introduced to new and different cultures. East Lancashire is home to many south Asian communities, especially Pakistani and Indian people. These communities tend to cluster in certain pockets or areas of towns, so they can be close by their family and friends.

Seeing inside the home of a Pakistani family in the 1970s was so interesting and intriguing. I loved the aromas that drifted down the street as I approached the houses and the way old English homes had been transformed inside to remind the inhabitants of their roots abroad.

In those days many families would arrange straight-backed sofas around the outside of the rooms, so they could double as beds. I'd often be amazed that there were so many family members in one house: I recall several occasions where I learned from conversations that grandparents, aunties and children – sometimes up to ten people – all lived in a two-bedroomed terraced property.

I soon became aware of how close-knit these communities were, and how well they looked after each other, especially new mothers, who were encouraged to rest for forty days after the birth. It was so interesting to see the different rituals of this community.

There was a tradition for one of the elders of the family

to whisper in the ear of a newborn baby and kohl was used to paint around the baby's eyes, like eyeliner. As soon as possible after the birth the baby's head would be shaved, as the hair was considered unclean. At that time the majority of the south Asian women we cared for didn't want to breastfeed their baby for the first three days, as they considered the colostrum (first milk) to also be unclean. As English wasn't commonly spoken, I learned that it was very difficult to communicate and to offer advice or information. But we did the best we could.

During my community experience I also had the wonderful opportunity of caring for my elder sister Eileen who was at the time pregnant with her youngest child. Eileen was booked to have her baby under the care of her community midwife and as luck would have it Sister Quinn was the midwife attached to my sister's GP surgery.

When she went into labour, Sister Quinn or one of the other community midwives would be on call and would go into hospital with Eileen to care for her. Best of all, as I was the pupil midwife attached to Sister Quinn I would potentially be around too!

Eileen and I had talked about the possibility of this happening and I was very touched when she said that she would really like me to help her to give birth to her baby.

My sister's due date came and went, but a few mornings later, on a day where I was due to work a night shift on call with Sister Quinn, Eileen started to have little niggles.

When she called to say her labour was starting, I was so thrilled. I tried not to get too excited as at this stage it could still have been a false alarm but Eileen promised to keep busy and that she would let me know how she was.

She phoned me a few times throughout the day to say little else had happened, but then, later, as I was sat with Paul in the staff residence, I got a call from her.

'I think I'm in labour,' she said. 'I'm coming in!'

As soon as I put the receiver down the call from Sister Quinn came, so I dashed across the hospital grounds to the maternity unit.

Arriving at the delivery suite I chose a suitable room for Eileen with Sister Quinn and we started to prepare things.

When Eileen arrived with her husband Denis, she was obviously in labour. 'Oh Sheena!' she whimpered, 'I don't like this.'

'You'll be fine!' I said, hugging her, and into the room we went.

So following procedure I faced the unpleasant task of shaving my sister. Well, Eileen may have been prepared to grin and bear that but when it came to the enema it was a whole different story. By now her contractions were coming thick and fast and as I began to funnel the liquid Eileen started to struggle.

'Stop it! Stop it!' she told me. I was really distressed to see how uncomfortable she was so I did something I'd never done before – I poured the liquid down the sink.

With the procedures complete (well, almost!) I led Eileen to the labour room where I would help Sister Quinn deliver the newest addition to our family.

I had a lot of experience by this stage but as a pupil I was still under the jurisdiction of my senior, the trained midwife.

I was pleased about this, as caring for a family member can be tricky. While it is an amazing and incredibly privileged position to be in, my emotions were clearly running high and at times I had to keep reminding myself that I had a professional accountability despite the family relationship.

For the next three hours I carefully looked after Eileen with the help of Denis, who was in the room and supporting her lovingly. When Eileen started to push, the excitement in the room increased tenfold.

'Come on, love, you are doing well!' Denis encouraged, as I concentrated on cradling the baby's head. The baby was born minutes later, with ease.

Scooping up the new arrival I looked up at Eileen with tears in my eyes. 'IT'S A GIRL!' I cried jubilantly.

Eileen and Denis already had two boys, Dominic and Daniel, and I knew Eileen secretly wanted a daughter. Scanning wasn't available in Burnley in the early 1970s and therefore she had no idea up until now.

'A GIRL? A GIRL? Oh Denis, it's a GIRL!' Eileen shouted. Denis was hugging her and crying, and Eileen wouldn't believe it until she saw for herself.

Before I passed my niece over to Eileen it was normal procedure to insert a tube into the baby's mouth or nostrils that was attached to a plastic gadget to clear the baby's airways (another practice now abolished). Eileen's baby didn't really need it but as the tears streamed down my face it was clear I couldn't see properly to do it.

'Stop crying, Murray!' Sister Quinn barked at me.

'Sorry,' I muttered, wiping away the tears and taking a big breath to compose myself. She was absolutely right.

Crying wasn't doing any good; I needed to concentrate. But it was just such a wonderful experience to help deliver my sister's baby and something I'll never forget.

All done, I passed the baby over to Eileen and Denis, who smothered her in kisses and wept. They called their new daughter Francesca. Ever since that moment I have felt a special bond with Francesca, who recently gave birth to the first baby of her own.

With Eileen and Denis head-over-heels with their beautiful daughter, Sister Quinn and I cleared everything away and headed off to make tea and toast.

Sweetly, Sister Quinn took me off to have a little chat about Francesca's birth.

'I can't believe that I have been so lucky,' I told her.

The following morning, after all the necessary checks had been carried out, Eileen and Denis took Francesca home to meet her brothers, Dominic and Daniel. Sister Quinn and I called in to make sure they were fine and we gave Eileen and Francesca a physical check.

We went back later in the evening to check again, which was the usual process when a woman went home after six hours. After that I visited my sister each day with Sister Quinn, and felt incredibly proud.

Unfortunately, Francesca developed severe jaundice a few days later and had to be admitted back into the maternity unit, causing Eileen and Denis much worry. Francesca's bilirubin levels were alarmingly high, right on the border of her needing an exchange blood transfusion. High bilirubin levels are dangerous and I was sick with worry, as I knew they could cause a type of brain damage called kernicterus.

Francesca was admitted to the special care baby unit (now called the neonatal intensive care unit) and throughout the day and night repeated blood checks were done while Eileen and Denis waited in anguish. Eventually the levels started to drop and Francesca was out of danger. We all started to relax a little although Francesca still had to be monitored closely. Thankfully with each day she improved and was eventually allowed to go home.

My year of training soon passed and once more a major examination loomed.

I revised whenever I could and Paul was very supportive, testing me at every opportunity and consequently becoming quite knowledgeable himself in the process. He now tells everyone he should have a qualification too.

The viva (oral exam) was the hardest and involved a senior midwifery manager and an obstetrician interviewing each candidate and giving them a pass or fail.

During my viva once again my nerves took over and when I entered the room my mouth wouldn't move! I did eventually answer all their questions and described what I would do in the scenarios they presented me with. To my utter joy I passed.

My written exam proved equally difficult, with three papers lasting four hours in total. I then had a torturous eight-week wait until the letter arrived with my overall result. I'd passed and was now a qualified midwife! The whole family celebrated with me, especially Paul.

Paul and I were now in the midst of planning our wedding for June 1978 just after my results came through and prior to our big day I briefly moved back home. As Paul helped me move my worldly possessions out of Bennett Johns House, Kate the Scottish cleaner was there to see me off.

Giving me a hug she turned to Paul and said, 'I'll miss seeing you climbing out of Sheena's window!' Oh dear, she knew all along. Good old Kate.

The build-up to my wedding was a very exciting time for me with plenty of planning and preparation. By now Paul and I had our small house in Burnley and had been saving hard to furnish it. I hadn't been in a position to do extra shifts but saved every spare penny towards our 'house fund'.

Meanwhile the midwives on the ward had also been busy planning and sprang their very own pre-wedding celebration on me. It involved putting me fully clothed in a bath, then adorning me with a handmade paper wedding dress, sitting me on a trolley and parading me round all the wards. The new mothers loved it and joined in the high spirits.

Our wedding day soon dawned, and as my father and I travelled to the Catholic church in the taxi, Dad held my hand and smiled at me all the way. He looked so proud and I know he felt very emotional escorting his fifth, and final, daughter down the aisle.

Seeing Paul smiling at me at the top of the aisle was wonderful and the whole service was so moving. Throughout the service my sister Lynne, who had a beautiful voice, played guitar and led the singing.

I spent the entire evening reception feeling so happy and dancing the night away.

The next day we headed off to Wales for our honeymoon, camping in a small tent. It rained so hard that we came home on day three! Not that we minded – it was just so exciting to be in our own house from then on and to begin our new life together.

However, despite our newlywed elation, we also had to learn how to actually live together for the first time, which wasn't always easy. I can remember one day off when I lovingly attempted to make Paul spaghetti bolognese for when he got home from work. I made miles too much, using a whole packet of spaghetti, but was so proud even though there were mountains of food on the table.

Yet Paul was shocked when he saw it and it showed in his voice.

'*How* much have you made?' he said.

I'd been expecting an 'oooh, how lovely', or maybe even a 'thank you'.

So I was left offended. In fact I was so cross that I picked the whole pan of sauce up and threw it in the bin.

This in turn angered Paul, who retaliated by throwing my spaghetti in the bin.

We argued for a moment, then fell about laughing – before heading out for a meal!

I returned to work as Mrs Byrom, which was strange but also nice. Now fully qualified, my uniform was pale blue, with white piping round the open-necked collar. I also wore a lacy starched cap and a pale blue belt with an antique silver buckle that my mum bought me.

Now a bona fide midwife I continued to deliver babies and even got to mentor pupil midwives too! I loved it.

Then in March 1979 to my absolute delight I discovered I was pregnant. I was twenty-four and had been married for nine months. Having witnessed the sheer joy of birth within my family and as a midwife, I couldn't wait to have my own little brood. Paul and I used to spend lots of time with my sisters who had children and we were particularly close to Anne and Eileen's little girls, Maria and Francesca. We were very keen to start a family, so when the nurse at the GP surgery handed me the slip that said 'positive', it was a very emotional moment. I immediately rushed home to tell Paul who was completely over the moon too.

I may have been on cloud nine at the news of my pregnancy but soon I was also hugging the toilet bowl. Unfortunately from early in my pregnancy I was plagued with horrendous morning sickness. I felt dreadful, like I was dying! I was working on the delivery suite at the time so found my sickness extremely debilitating.

I can recall one particularly bad day when I was caring for a woman in labour. I'd hoped my nausea would lessen, as it normally did as the day went on, but on this particular afternoon it was still there with a vengeance.

Normally I would have asked a colleague to take over from me or help out, but it was a busy shift and everyone was tied up. I had also built up a close relationship with the woman I was caring for and seeing as she was getting to the final stages I really wanted to see the birth through.

I'd already left her for brief periods to take a sip of water in an attempt to relieve the intense sickness but eventually I had to leave abruptly to vomit.

Luckily I was only out of the room for a few minutes and

immediately felt better when I returned – just in time to catch her baby.

Apart from the sickness, being pregnant while I worked on the delivery ward was a lovely experience – not least as the women I cared for loved chatting to me about my pregnancy and giving me advice!

As my pregnancy advanced and my bump grew I was proud as punch. Seeing other parents happily starting their family had made me broody. But I also found it hard physically as time went on. Running around on the delivery suite wasn't easy, especially when it got busy. My fingers swelled up, I felt tired as the shift went on and I struggled bending over. I was always glad to get my feet up at the end of the day. Thankfully I didn't really feel more emotional than usual, and I relaxed as much as I could by reading, walking and knitting.

I also spent lots of time with my sisters Eileen and Anne. Susan lived in Surrey at this stage and was also pregnant (with her second child), so we used to chat on the phone and compare notes.

Back home our family were experiencing worrying times. In May 1978 Dad had suffered a stroke whilst he was doing some work for a friend. A year later his health worsened significantly and he started to go downhill.

When he became critically ill, Mum, my sisters and I took turns nursing him at home and sitting with him all night. We were all so sad, especially Mum, and with Susan and I both pregnant it was a real strain. The nights were long and poor Dad was very sick. We knew he was going to die.

One evening I had just left him and gone home to bed, when Paul came to wake me. He was crying.

'I'm sorry, Sheena,' he said. 'Your dad has died.'

I jumped out of bed and drove round to Mum's as quickly as I could. One by one, members of the family arrived and we cried together. We'd known it was coming but yet a world without Dad seemed inconceivable. We had no idea how we could even begin to fill the void in our lives.

I was five months' pregnant and so it was terribly upsetting for me that my father hadn't lived to meet my baby, and I knew my sister Susan felt the same. Dad had known that he was going to have more grandchildren but sadly never saw our baby girls – Jane, born first, and Anna, born three days after her.

It was hard to go back to work feeling so sad but keeping busy did help to distract me from my grief. Then of course the time came for me to leave my job and concentrate on my baby.

I was seven months' pregnant by now and although maternity leave was an option for me I wanted to be a full-time mum to my child and not to worry about working. Paul and I had discussed it at length and although it would be a struggle without a second salary, we felt we could manage.

When the time came for me to have my baby I was giddy with excitement. I didn't know what sex the baby was but Paul and I really wanted a little girl because of the time spent with our nieces.

I wasn't worried or anxious about giving birth. My mum and my sisters often talked about the pain of labour as being difficult, but with a positive slant. 'There's always an end to it,' they said. 'And it's a wonderful relief when the baby is born!' It was very matter-of-fact in my family: women had babies and that was that. Mum always said that it was an amazing experience and I believed her.

And of course while I had seen women give birth after long, hard labours, I'd also witnessed the ecstatic elation when the baby was born.

Being so knowledgeable about what happens to women's bodies physically during labour, it was strange actually going through it for myself. But, in a way, knowing what was happening made me feel relaxed. It was reassuring to have my colleagues caring for me as I trusted them and felt in safe hands.

I started having contractions a few days after my due date and went into hospital for a check. My colleague Margaret, one of the senior midwives, examined me and I was disappointed to learn nothing much was happening. 'What do you want to do?' she enquired. 'Go home or have your waters broken?'

This procedure was routinely done in the 1970s but in hindsight I regret my decision to go ahead. Now I understand how potentially dangerous it is to rush nature, especially when there is no reason to and all is going well. But at the time I was impatient.

I was taken into a delivery room where one of the senior doctors performed the task. It was extremely uncomfortable but I concentrated on the fact my baby was going to be with me soon. No such luck. My labour turned out to be long and hard, most likely because I wasn't really ready to give birth.

The progress wasn't good and after many hours had passed and I had become exhausted, the doctors decided that I needed syntocinon in a drip to speed things up.

Syntocinon is a synthetic hormone that stimulates contractions but these are much stronger than the natural type and begin suddenly, rather than building up at a gentle pace. Consequently the body hasn't got time to adjust and the natural pain-relieving hormones – the endorphins – fail to kick in properly. As I was hit by contractions of juggernaut proportions I really started to feel distressed.

I had several 'shots' of pethidine to help me but it just made me drowsy, and meanwhile the contractions were relentless. I felt exhausted, dazed and overwhelmed, and Paul, who'd remained by my side, was getting more and more worried.

Eventually Margaret, my midwife, suggested that I should see a new locum (relief) consultant obstetrician who was working that day. Apparently he had worked in London where epidurals were performed and he said I would be able to have one if I wanted.

In 1979 epidurals were not common and the only person I'd heard who'd had one was Cilla Black! They certainly weren't used when I was a student midwife. Instead women were supported through their labours by the staff – a practice I wholeheartedly believed in. But here I was, exhausted, distressed and not really in a position to think straight. I didn't really like the sound of it but I would have accepted anything (a limb amputation even) if it took my pain away. So I agreed.

Paul was horrified and went to call my family. My sister Anne, who was a nurse, immediately called the delivery suite to find out more information. As she was lucid and not in labour she realised that my decision was perhaps not the wisest one but by then I'd already consented.

When the doctor came to do the procedure I was told to lie on my side and bend my knees up as far as I could towards my chest. It was very uncomfortable. Meanwhile he tried to insert the needle into my back. He was clearly having problems and it took him a long time, but the midwives had no choice but to trust him as they had never seen this procedure before.

Whenever I recall this moment I do not fail to cringe when I think I let a doctor who was probably untrained in the technique (it is anaesthetic doctors who perform epidurals) mess with my spine.

When the ordeal was finally over the doctor and Margaret turned me over and waited for my next contraction.

'It's not working!' I cried, as a wave of pain hit me once more.

Although the doctor said it could take a while, the relief never came.

'I need to do it again,' he concluded, and once again I was turned on my side to be prodded and poked. Another fifteen minutes passed (Paul told me later) and he believed it had been a success. Once more I was turned on to my back and the team waited with bated breath.

'No,' I cried. 'It's not worked!' By this stage I was desperate so I moved on to my side with help for a third time and after yet another attack on my spine the anaesthetic finally worked. The relief came approximately ten minutes after the procedure and I relaxed – but not for long.

'I think I want to push!' I declared. Margaret checked me and my baby was indeed coming. I didn't feel an overwhelming urge to push (like I did later with my other children) but I did feel something strange happening and instinctively knew that my baby was going to be born.

A few minutes later, Margaret scooped up a tiny darkhaired baby. 'It's a girl!' she said, handing her over to me. Although I was utterly exhausted my eyes immediately scanned her gorgeous little face. My heart surged, and I cried. She was just perfect and Paul and I wept tears of happiness. We named our little beauty Anna Catherine Byrom. I couldn't stop looking at her blinking sleepily in my arms or listening to her making her soft baby gurgles. I held her close, talked to her and marvelled at her little button nose and tiny fingers and toes. I'd seen new mums going gooey over their babies time and again and now it all made perfect sense. The rush of love I felt towards Anna was just incredible.

After loads of cuddles and a cup of tea, I had a go at breastfeeding. Thankfully I found it straightforward and used the skills I learned as a midwife to help me get started. It was slightly painful but I got through it to find it very rewarding.

Leaving me to rest, Paul kissed both Anna and me on the forehead and went off to collect his mother so she could be introduced to her first grandchild.

By now I'd been taken to the postnatal ward and was just in heaven with my new baby. As my mum and sisters had said, all thoughts of labour pain were long forgotten and I just remember absolute bliss.

There was one slight problem though: my epidural was still going strong and I was effectively paralysed from the waist down. I couldn't feel anything so I couldn't walk or go to the toilet. It was really problematic as no one was trained in epidurals and the midwives didn't know what to do with me.

The midwife told me they needed to take Anna to the nursery for the night, as I couldn't care for her due to my paralysis.

'No,' I argued. 'I don't want her to leave me. I don't want them to take her.'

I loved her so much, but the midwife was adamant that it was safer and to my utter dismay they took her out the room for 'an hour'.

I must have dozed off when I heard a baby crying. It just sparked such an extreme reaction in me. Desperate to get to my baby I tried to get out of bed but my legs still weren't working so I fell on the floor. One of the midwives found me there crying – awful considering that these members of staff were all my colleagues and friends.

'You have to bring my baby back,' I begged them. 'You'll just have to help me to get her out the cot.' So Anna was missing for two hours but after that I never let her out my sight.

Afterwards I felt annoyed that the situation had happened. I had never wanted Anna to go. I know I was very possessive with her, really believing I was the only one that could care for her properly, but I loved being a new mum and thoroughly enjoyed the special moments we spent together, such as feeding in the night, just the two of us. I didn't mind the lack of sleep and loved her smell, her breath and her sweet little face.

Back home, adjusting to life as a new mum, I also had some hair-raising moments. I can remember one day when Anna was about three months old and I put her in her car seat and set off to my mum's house in the next town. I was singing songs to her and glancing in the rear mirror to see if she was OK, when suddenly to my horror I saw that the car seat was empty. My stomach churning with shock I pulled up and scrambled into the back of the car. There she was in the footwell, gurgling, smiling and playing with her fingers, not a care in the world! I'd forgotten to put the car seat straps on and she'd slipped down!

This was not the only occasion I thought she'd vanished. I used to have vivid anxiety dreams where I'd be convinced she'd disappeared from the crib next to our bed. One night when she was six weeks old I woke up in a terrible state.

'She's gone!' I screamed, causing Paul to shoot out the bed.

'Find her, find her,' I begged. Then as I heard Paul careering around the house I spied her fast asleep in her crib. I just burst into tears. I thought I'd lost the plot!

Mum was a great support to me, and my sisters too. They offered plenty of advice, telling me it was normal to worry and that I would learn to be less anxious as time went on. Having these experiences definitely helped me in the future as a midwife when I supported mothers who felt anxious and worried after the birth of their baby. Having been through it myself I could really empathise.

It did get easier and gradually I learned to relax. By the time Anna was four months old I had settled in to a lovely routine with my little family and seeing Anna growing day by day was a real joy.

Then, to my utter shock, I fell pregnant again.

Chapter 6

Standing in the chemists, I stared in horror at the piece of paper in my hand.

'PREGNANT' it read, revealing the results of the test I had just taken. Bursting into tears I immediately ran out the door, leaving a perplexed-looking Paul with Anna in her pram.

It was when I started to feel sick in the mornings again that I'd first begun to worry. Anna was four months old and I was still wandering around in my maternity dresses having lost none of my pregnancy weight.

I was breastfeeding and foolishly thought I couldn't get pregnant but when I'd started to feel nauseous Paul had duly accompanied me to the local chemists to find out.

Now he was having to chase his distraught wife down the street trying his hardest not to mow down passing pedestrians with Anna's pram.

'Sheena! Sheena!' he yelled. When he eventually caught up with me Anna's hair was stood on end.

'Come on, Sheena,' he said, rubbing my back as I sobbed. 'It's brilliant news!'

He was right, it was wonderful, but I think at the time I

was just overwhelmed, wondering how I could possibly cope with another baby. I'd only just got a grip of my worrying with Anna.

As it happened, my second pregnancy was lovely. I wasn't as sick, and, as is usual with second pregnancies, I didn't have time to fuss so much.

But we did need somewhere new to live, not just for our expanding brood but also so I could be nearer to Mum.

So when I was six months' pregnant we moved house to Clitheroe, the historical market town where I'd lived as a child, which was about a mile from Mum's home in a small village called West Bradford.

Our new home was a large old Victorian terrace on Pimlico Road. We loved it immediately, and as the previous elderly owner had died suddenly, we were able to move in fairly quickly as we had sold our property in Burnley. But our new home was large and in an expensive area, so we were forced to undertake a huge mortgage to pay for it. We could cover it with Paul's job as a toolmaker, but then we had the most dreadful shock when Paul was made redundant. To add to our problems interest rates started to soar.

Although Paul immediately got a new, more secure job, it wasn't as well paid. At a stretch we could just about cover the mortgage but not much else.

Mum was a lifesaver, helping us as much as she could by donating meat and other provisions. She also baked for us and invited us round to hers for meals. It was so hard. Even buying milk, bread and other basics was a real struggle.

We also had some really good neighbours and I can remember one particular friend called Christine who knew about our situation and called over one day with some meat she'd taken out of her freezer. Her kindness was very touching and I'll never forget her.

For several months, right up until after our second child was born, we had a very stressful time living hand to mouth. Although Paul thought all would be well in the end, I worried about the future.

Moving to a new area meant a change of family doctor and likewise the midwives who were caring for me during my pregnancy changed too.

The Clitheroe community midwife was called Pauline Quinn and I liked her instantly. During our initial meeting she took a medical history from me and chatted to me about where I wanted to have my baby. I didn't know it then, but Pauline was to become a huge influence in my career and a real inspiration to me. Thirty years on Pauline is now one of my dear friends.

Meanwhile I had a baby to give birth to. It was Boxing Day 1980 and we were eating dinner at my sister Lynne's house when my labour started. Paul drove me to Burnley where I was lucky enough to have the same midwife – Margaret – who'd helped me during Anna's birth. Despite being my community midwife, Pauline would only attend if I'd opted for a home birth.

Even though Anna's birth had been long and hard, I wasn't too worried about the labour this time. I was optimistic that the second time round it would be better and

I was now very excited at the prospect of meeting my new baby.

Again, we didn't know the sex; it still wasn't offered as an option in those days, but we wouldn't have wanted to spoil the surprise anyway.

My labour was actually just as hard as the first, but much shorter, and because I didn't have an epidural I was able to really experience the wonderful moment of birth.

Through strong contractions I pushed out our baby. I'd just got my breath back when Paul looked up at me with tears in his eyes. 'It's a boy!' he said.

I scooped our son up immediately and together Paul and I examined our little man for the very first time.

'I'd like to call him James after my dad,' I said. Paul nodded in delighted agreement.

Our bouncing baby boy was so different to his sister. He seemed big and beautiful and had the most enormous mouth! We were thrilled, now proud parents to a boy and a girl – how lucky we were.

We snuggled him up and I gave him his first breastfeed. Margaret had informed us that our son weighed an impressive 9 lb 10 oz! Wow! He was going to need some filling.

This time I went home after about six hours as I felt so well and wanted to be with Anna who was still only fourteen months old. It was so special to be home with our little family at Christmas and we felt extremely lucky.

After James's birth my family gathered round to help. There was an abundance of home baking, hot meals and general support from my sisters and my mother.

I loved being a mum and remember those days with fondness. Admittedly it was hard with the two little ones but our biggest worry was the fact that money was still tight and the pressure to pay bills and live from day to day was stressful.

One day, when James was about four months old, my sister Anne called to say she'd spotted a job advert requesting midwives to work night duty (part- and full-time) at a maternity home called Bramley Meade, which was in Whalley, about four miles from Clitheroe.

Bramley Meade was a small maternity unit run by midwives and GPs that fell under the Blackburn group of hospitals. I knew of it as my sister Anne had worked there on nights as a nurse when her children were young and some of my nieces and nephews were born there.

'Maybe you could work one night a week?' Anne suggested. 'I did that when my children were small and it really helped.' I hadn't planned on going back to work until my children were much older, but this seemed like a good opportunity as I'd heard it was a great place to work and it would help us to make ends meet.

I spoke to Paul at length about it when he came home from work and we agreed that if I could do a few hours there it would definitely boost our income. My family also offered to help out so I rang up and spoke to the senior midwife who invited me in the next day for an interview.

The next morning Mum popped round to look after Anna and James as I donned my smartest outfit and made my way to Bramley Meade.

The maternity unit was housed in a beautiful grand

mansion house set amongst pretty gardens and trees. It had once been home to a wealthy mill owner and his family, and was converted to a maternity home in 1950.

There was a lodge where the caretaker lived and a boat house that was boarded up. The building was imposing but full of character.

My interview was conducted by Mrs Heyes, a nursing officer who'd come from Blackburn's Queens Park Hospital to interview me. It wasn't exactly in-depth and was very informal. Mrs Heyes asked me a few questions about my experience as a midwife and explained that they had decided to increase the number of staff at the home to ensure two midwives worked every night.

I mentioned that I would probably only want to work one night a week – so a twelve-hour shift – although I might be able to increase to two nights a week in the future. I loved midwifery and would be pleased to be back at work in this brilliant environment but I had to consider my family. I didn't want to do any more as I was still breastfeeding. But working one shift a week simply meant I'd have enough money to buy food.

'You can work as many or as few hours as you'd like,' she agreed. 'So can you start tonight?' They were clearly desperate for staff!

'Um, not tonight,' I said apologetically. 'I have a small baby and need to make some arrangements, but maybe next week,' I said.

So it was quickly agreed that I'd work one night a week.

Back home later in the day, Mum, Paul and I sat down and thrashed out the arrangements. It wasn't going to be easy with a fifteen-month-old and a baby. Paul started work at 6 a.m. each day and I wouldn't get home until 8 a.m. so Mum agreed to come and look after the children from 6 a.m. until 8 a.m. Once I got home she'd then stay on to keep an eye on them while I had a sleep. It was a massive sacrifice on her part but it was the only way we could have managed it.

When the time came for me to do my first night shift I had so many anxieties. The last thing I wanted to do was leave my tiny baby and I drove to work crying my eyes out. I'd left James some expressed breast milk but I was worried it wouldn't be enough. I was also worried about little Anna: how would she feel when I wasn't there in the morning? I felt like I was abandoning them. I was also anxious about my first shift. I'd be working with new staff under a different system and had no idea what would be expected of me. Like everywhere else I'd worked, Bramley Meade had its own hierarchical system and distinct culture.

My first night shift was a real eye-opener. I was welcomed by Sister Carla Gazzola, an Italian midwife who was to become my lifelong friend and also the midwife I chose to care for me when I had two further children.

Carla was single and lived at Bramley Meade in a suite of rooms. My first impression was that Carla was stern and very much 'in charge'. She was very formal and scared me slightly, although years later when I told her this she was shocked and upset as she really didn't intend to be!

Carla was quietly spoken and of course had an Italian accent. She had clear ideas of how she liked things to be done, and she made them known. I was to learn on that first night that Carla was a stickler for routine and when she was on duty we were to follow practice. For example, mothers quite rightly were the 'queens' and received the most wonderful attention. Drinks were to be given last thing at night (and then of course all night on demand), babies taken to the nursery at night, bins emptied, sterilising solutions changed – all before 11 p.m. Then it was lights out and whispers so as not to disturb the women. When I'd left Burnley the practice of taking babies away from their mothers at night was being phased out as it was recognised as being harmful. I was surprised to learn it was still standard procedure at Bramley. Mothers could keep their baby beside them overnight if they really wanted but I got the impression that many mothers reluctantly agreed to have their babies removed because they were worried that their child would disturb the other mothers who'd opted to sleep.

The nursery where the babies were taken was a former billiard room. There were hooks on the walls where the cues used to rest and the dark brown panelling helped to conjure up the picture of previous activities. The room was large and was accessed from the main foyer via a heavy wooden door with a glass panel at the top.

Each evening the babies would be wheeled into the room, and placed in a line. Unless a mother really protested the routine was set here too, and babies would be fed four hourly or pacified or given water if they woke up in between those times. I recall dummies being used, and if none were available staff would push cotton wool balls in a disposable teat and use that as a dummy! It was very rarely quiet in that nursery, as there was nearly always one baby crying.

Taking babies to the nursery whilst the mothers slept was all geared towards the needs of the mother – the women were tired and often exhausted and would sleep for long periods of time. But a newborn baby is biologically programmed to feed regularly and frequently, in small amounts, whenever he wants. The whole process is so alien to today's practice, where babies are fed on demand.

Women may have felt they were benefiting from a night's sleep but for those who were breastfeeding this presented a problem. As the babies weren't feeding during the night, many women used to wake up with exceptionally full and hard breasts. Often it would lead to an engorgement – where the breasts would swell and throb because not enough milk was being extracted by the baby – or even the painful infection mastitis.

Instead of thinking that perhaps something was physiologically wrong, we 'treated' the condition with something called breast binding. We'd fold a draw sheet in a particular way and wrap it around the woman's chest from back to front, pulling it as tight as we could and securing it with nappy pins. The women liked it because they said they felt comfortable but it was very time consuming. Really we should have encouraged and supported them to feed their babies more frequently but at the time breast binding was viewed as best and that was the way things were done.

Having all the babies in the nursery overnight occasionally led to embarrassing mix-ups. In the morning we would take the babies back to their mothers, which took a long time as there were women based upstairs and the lift was small, only fitting two cots and one staff member in at a time.

I can remember one awful morning when a mother called me over.

'Excuse me,' she said, ever so politely. 'The baby I gave you last night had a blue name band and this baby has a pink name band.' To this day I am not sure why she didn't say, 'This is a girl and I gave birth to a little boy!'

I tried not to let the alarm show on my face. Oh my goodness, it was the wrong baby. Who have I given her baby to? It was a very bad moment but thankfully I quickly tracked her baby down and put the situation right again. When I discussed this hazard with my old colleagues recently, many of them admitted they had done the same thing during the years that babies were separated from their mothers. Indeed, one of the auxiliary nurses that worked at Bramley Meade for more than two decades told me that before I worked there staff used to carry all the babies back to their mothers in their arms and several times she gave a mum the wrong baby. Thank goodness the risk of this happening today is minimised as a baby rarely leaves his or her mother's side.

On my first night, after the handover from the day staff had been given, Carla instructed Jane, a staff nurse on duty, to show me round. Seeing as there was no one in labour that night Jane was able to fill me in on all the routines I would need to adhere to.

As she gave me the guided tour I was suddenly aware of how huge Bramley Meade was. As I followed Jane I found myself mesmerised by the building's previous grandeur, not least the austere staircase sweeping from the entrance hall to the next floor, the Italian marble pillars in the foyer and the beautiful stained glass windows.

The house also had an attic that used to be the servants' quarters and an enormous cellar. To get to the cellar you had to go through a door opposite the manager's office. As you crept down the steps it was dry but dark and dingy. I was completely startled when, at the bottom, Jane pointed to a door and said, 'That's the mortuary.' I hadn't expected to find that in the building. She went on to explain that thankfully the room was not used very often but she believed it had been used in the past to put babies in until the undertaker came.

There was also a room full of old maternity records, with details of the labours and births that had taken place over the years at Bramley Meade.

Next door was an incinerator room, which I was dismayed to learn I'd have to visit morning and night to deposit the plastic bin bags full of rubbish. The laundry also got sorted down there. Outside the incinerator room was an assortment of aerosol cans and other items that were all black and damaged.

'What are all those for?' I asked Jane.

'Mr Wilson, the caretaker, leaves items there to remind us we shouldn't put them in the rubbish bins,' she said. 'He goes mad if we forget.'

I found it all very interesting but slightly intimidating.

At Burnley I'd had the luxury of a centralised sterilisation department where dirty instruments used in the delivery packs and for suturing were sent to be thoroughly cleaned, packaged up and sent back as good as new. However, at Bramley Meade we had to do this ourselves using old-fashioned vessels and machines. We even had huge tongs called cheadles, that looked like salad servers, to handle the instruments and keep them sterile, which was quite a palaver. The clean instruments were then stored in a special solution until needed and although it was everyone's responsibility to ensure there was enough apparatus for the shift, the task usually fell on the support staff, who were very proficient at the procedure.

Upstairs on the ground level was an enormous kitchen, similar to those you'd see in a Victorian house – very like *Upstairs, Downstairs*. There was a huge oven range with large kettles that were on the boil all day and all night to provide hot water for the drinks for the women. Every so often a member of staff would have to check they hadn't boiled dry.

On the wall above the door was the remnants of a bell system left over from when Bramley was a private residence and the staff still used it.

The mothers had their meals downstairs in the dining room, apart from those who'd just had babies who were served in bed. Meanwhile the staff used to dine together in the sitting room and when finished with their first course they'd ring the bell and a waitress would come and clear the plates. This was not the norm for the NHS and the staff felt very cared for!

This perk was stopped a few years later but it must have been nice for the staff while it lasted. Of course during the night we didn't have that luxury, although on some evenings we were lucky enough to enjoy the wonderful cooking of Sister Gazzola.

Carla was a brilliant cook, and when she was working she'd disappear into the big kitchen at about 11 p.m., when all the mothers and babies were settled, and set to work at the range. She'd concoct the most amazing soups using herbs and spices and leftovers she'd gathered. I can still remember the glorious smell wafting through before the feast appeared. She'd also pick weeds from the garden at certain times of the year and after carefully cleaning them would mix them with eggs and make us fritters. We loved them. Carla retired back to Italy in 1990 and although we are still close friends I miss her so much. When I see those particular weeds on country roadsides around Lancashire I always think of the food Carla made for us and the smells and tastes she introduced us to!

After a few weeks at Bramley I got into a little routine. The day of my shift I'd look after the children in the day and try and rest as much as I could. Mum would come round before I went to work to allow me a little time to sleep but because I was breastfeeding I didn't really get much.

After a hard but wonderfully satisfying night caring for mothers and babies and fighting fatigue – it was very hard as I felt extreme tiredness when it was my responsibility to be alert – I'd drive home to find James ravenous, and Mum trying to pacify him.

Mum would pass him to me and he'd latch on immediately and guzzle away. I used to lie on the bed and fall asleep while I was feeding him so Mum would stay close to me and gently lift him away once he was done. She would then stay around most of the day looking after the children while I slept.

It was quite a journey. Now I am older I often think, 'How on earth did I do all that?' Like many midwives who work when they have a young family, it seems like I did the impossible but at the time I just took it in my stride. I had so many responsibilities. I was only twenty-three and we had a huge mortgage, two children and I worked as a midwife at night. In the end I stayed at Bramley Meade for eight years doing one or two nights a week, right through from 1981 when James was a baby until the unit closed in 1989.

It was quite a significant time in my life. As a young mum myself I really felt connected to childbearing women, and I felt I had an intuition about what they needed.

However, when I went back to work after having James it was really too early. There was no denying it was quite an unnatural situation dealing with other babies when, perhaps, I should have been at home with my own.

In the early days I had a real problem as every time I went near a baby my milk 'let down', or in other words I started to lactate. This is a natural response and most breastfeeding mothers will find that when they touch or see another baby then more milk comes. But with twenty or more babies to deal with my breasts were on overdrive!

I can remember one particular night when I was helping a woman to breastfeed. Her baby was in the nursery and she had asked to be woken to feed her baby when he stirred. As I assisted this mother I bent over to help her to position her baby at her breast.

Suddenly I realised she seemed a bit distracted.

'Are you OK?' I asked.

'My knees are wet,' she said, looking puzzled.

Looking down, I immediately realised the problem.

'I'm so sorry,' I told her. 'It's my breast milk!'

Well, that took some explaining.

Bramley Meade was a maternity home for women who were considered to be 'low risk', meaning they had no complications or expected complications. GPs would 'book' them in only if they were deemed 'suitable'.

There were no resident doctors although local GPs could come for the birth and to see women afterwards. There was limited medical equipment, apart from resuscitation apparatus, and women who came there were encouraged and supported to have their babies naturally.

Women giving birth at Bramley were very privileged: the attention they received was second to none and they got one-on-one care. When a woman arrived in labour I rarely left her side. In the main I'd sit and support her throughout the night as she found her most comfortable space in one of the two labour rooms and manoeuvered herself into a position that best worked for her.

As well as catching babies we looked after women who'd been transferred from Queens Park Hospital after Caesarean sections or instrumental births, i.e. ones in which forceps or a ventouse (a vacuum device) were used to assist the delivery of a baby.

Women, brought from Queens Park by ambulance on a daily basis, were often exhausted when they arrived, having just come from a busy hospital where the care and attention wasn't as focused. When they arrived they'd often seem happy and relieved thanks to the good reputation Bramley Meade had in the community for providing excellent support.

Being in such a wonderful environment was lovely for the midwives too and I felt like I really built up my skills at Bramley Meade. I learned to use my eyes and my hands to ensure mothers and babies were safe and I enjoyed working in surroundings where I could give women enough time to nurture them.

I loved witnessing the closeness of women with their partners and never failed to be awed by the immense pleasure of mothers as they saw their baby for the first time.

In the less busy moments when all the women were settled, we would sit in the staff sitting room and read or knit. Carla Gazzola was one of the key knitters at Bramley Meade. She had this lovely French knitting pattern for baby booties, which looked like proper little shoes, and she would add tiny pompoms to the top of them. She used to rustle up hundreds of pairs of these booties, which she'd sell to the mothers for about £1 a pair to raise money for the charity Save the Children. They were so popular that we used to take orders. Carla could knit at an impressive speed, often clocking up eight pairs of booties a night.

The wool was made up of odds and ends that Carla had sourced cheaply from a lady called Jill who had a wool shop in Whalley Village, and often patients themselves would send in bundles of their leftover yarn. It was like a cottage industry! I think this was perhaps unethical (we are certainly not allowed to sell anything to patients these days) but it was so special, and it connected mothers and midwives with a charity, in addition to enhancing the babies' wardrobes! My knitting skills were inspired by family tradition and by Carla's skill and patience. We would share patterns and during the wee small hours of the morning when all was still in the home she would give me tips on how to do unusual stitches. As I sat knitting for Anna and James, Carla would ask me about my children and then surprise me a week later with a small garment she had made for one of them as a gift. She did this for other staff members too and was very generous.

Chapter 7

The stories of what went on at Bramley Meade in its early days as a maternity unit were told and retold during the intimate night shifts when staff worked closely together for twelve hours.

I loved hearing the stories from years gone by and was very intrigued by the tales of old practices and how things had changed.

Some of the staff remembered the time when babies were kept in the nursery at all times, day and night, except for feeding times when they were taken back to their mothers.

Fathers were allowed to see their babies at visiting time – but could only catch a glimpse through the glass panel in the nursery door as a member of staff held their baby up to the glass.

It was clear that practices were constantly evolving and the rules often changed depending on which senior midwife was in charge and how 'traditional' her approach was.

I might have been able to have Paul by my side for Anna and James's births but during my early years at Bramley Meade husbands were generally sent home once they'd dropped off their wives. Some of the men seemed more than relieved to disappear and I don't recall any woman telling me she was unhappy with the situation. However, everyone had an opinion and it was funny listening to the contradicting views as they were debated in the staff room.

'Men don't help anyway,' one senior midwife declared. 'It's better that they go home.'

However, times were changing and Bramley Meade was about to enter a period where practices would be revolutionised and the maternity unit as a whole would take on a very modern approach.

These changes were spearheaded by Pauline Quinn, the midwife who had cared for me when I'd been pregnant with James. After working in the community for many years, Pauline had been promoted and arrived at Bramley Meade as a nursing officer.

A lovely lady, who hailed from Liverpool, Pauline had radical ideas for the way maternity care should move forward. Over the next four years she led dramatic changes in the way things were done at Bramley.

One of her initial changes was to invite husbands to stay with their wives during labour if they wanted to. From then on I have vivid memories of men supporting their wives in labour and through the births of their babies with such tenderness.

It clearly mattered to these women that their husbands were there with them and it was a real joy to see the reaction of these proud new fathers in the moments when their daughter or son was born.

Of course I also recall times when well-meaning husbands or partners have actually added to the drama . . .

I can remember one warm, humid night in the labour room where a woman was using every last ounce of energy to push her baby out. We'd shut all the windows to avoid being besieged by night buzzards and moths and the poor mum was hot, sweaty and thoroughly exhausted.

I was beside her, encouraging her to keep pushing, when suddenly I noticed her husband slipping slowly down the side of the bed, banging his head on a radiator in the process. Maureen, my midwife colleague, rushed to his side.

I was concentrating on helping the mother but glancing across I was alarmed to see he wasn't moving and had a graze on his head.

'He's out cold!' Maureen confirmed.

Just at that moment the baby's head started to emerge.

'Just leave him!' the mother screamed. 'He'll be all right!'

I carried on with the job at hand while Maureen quickly checked the unfortunate husband's breathing and pulse and propped a pillow under his head. She dashed back to assist just as the couple's baby was born.

Typically the husband came to just as we'd placed the tiny tot in his wife's arms.

'Oh, you've decided to join us, have you?' she remarked as he struggled to his feet in a confused fashion, rubbing his head.

Working under Mrs Quinn's reign was exciting as we all began to see the effect her changes were having on the care women received. Whilst the changes she instigated weren't always popular, they were always based on what she believed was best for both mothers and babies.

It was Mrs Quinn who introduced 'rooming in' to Bramley,

which meant babies were no longer taken away from their mothers at night and instead remained by their bedsides.

I found her work very inspiring and she became a huge role model for me. I liked the fact we were giving women 'choice' and that in every aspect of our work we were encouraged to support women to give birth in the way they wanted to.

Keen to promote normal birth, Mrs Quinn introduced a birthing stool that was designed to help women to have their baby naturally and also birth mats for women to use on the floor to adopt different positions. In the early 1980s this was considered very radical and in many ways she was before her time. Indeed some of the practices she introduced to the maternity home are still being implemented today in some units.

In addition to the birth aids, Mrs Quinn purchased a cassette tape player so women could bring in their favourite music to play whilst they were in labour.

To have music playing during labour was obviously beneficial for the parents but we loved it too. It clearly helped to create a more relaxing atmosphere and women often commented how familiar sounds helped to reduce some of their anxieties.

Personal tastes in music weren't always compatible, however, and I remember some rather bizarre choices of music. One couple brought in an unusual mix of American rock music that included 'Bat Out of Hell' by Meat Loaf.

I wouldn't exactly describe it as calming but there we were, rocking away as we rubbed her back and mopped her brow . . . it certainly kept us in rhythm!

Usually, the music chosen was of the more gentle variety, typically ballads or classical pieces. One particular birth stands out in my memory: Claire and Tim were having their first baby and Claire's labour was particularly long and hard.

Their chosen music was *The Four Seasons* by Vivaldi and I was totally amazed by the reaction Claire had to the music when it was playing.

She moved with it, swaying to the individual sounds of each track and smiling. When baby Olivia was born it was like a scene from a romantic movie. I was inspired by Claire's calmness and the love between the couple and their new baby was palpable.

When I told the couple afterwards how much I had enjoyed caring for them and how wonderful I thought baby Olivia's birth was, they gave me the tapes.

I still see them from time to time in Clitheroe and now whenever I hear *The Four Seasons* I think of them and their very special birth.

As far as peaceful surroundings went the grounds of Bramley Meade, with its oak trees and beautiful gardens, could not have been more perfect. Each year as spring arrived, the night staff looked forward to the dawn chorus as birdsong signalled a new day – meaning that the chance to sleep was near!

At certain times of the year as dusk fell, we would be aware of the large colony of bats that lived in the old roof space of the house. Although we couldn't see them clearly as we gazed out from the brightly lit labour room, hundreds of swarming and swooping bats was undoubtedly an eerie sight.

Often when I was helping with a labour I'd catch one out of the corner of my eye. It was really quite off-putting. Likewise it hardly brought comfort to anxious husbands pacing the floors as they waited for their firstborn to arrive. Indeed the ghoulish sight of black creatures flying past were often marked with cries of, 'Oh my God, what was that?'

But over time I came to get used to them – or so I thought.

One night I was sat in the sitting room chatting with a midwife friend when there was a knock on the door. When I went to investigate I found a woman in her dressing gown.

'Sorry, I don't mean to disturb you,' she said. 'But there is a bat hanging from the curtain in my room.'

My first thought was that she'd left her baby to come and tell us. So hurrying out the sitting room I quickly walked with her back to her room.

As I walked into the area it was a struggle not to scream. There, hanging upside down from the curtain rail of her bed, was a bat, about the size of a small rat.

'I'm so sorry but I think we need to move you and your baby out of this room,' I told her, attempting to keep my voice calm and quiet and at the same time thanking my lucky stars that she was the only woman in the room.

Gathering up her belongings gingerly so as not to disturb the bat, I bundled her and her baby out of the room, shutting the door firmly behind us.

After I'd got her comfortable next door I scribbled a note to Mr Wilson, the handyman, to tell him the tale, and asking him to get rid of it. My, if this happened today there would need to be a full investigation and a 'risk analysis' report just in case an 'adverse event' had happened.

The next day I'd forgotten all about the bat. I was too busy immersing myself in family life. I did sometimes find it hard juggling work and home life, but thankfully there were playgroups and Paul and I got lots of help from family and friends.

We were always busy and had full lives. We didn't have a garden so at weekends or when I was off we would always be picnicking somewhere. Brimham Rocks in Yorkshire was our favourite haunt. Then when finances improved we had lovely holidays on a budget, camping in Padstow in Cornwall at first and then eventually progressing to France.

We also visited the family of Genevieve, my pen friend from school. The tiredness was ongoing but I used to go to bed early!

Thankfully my marriage with Paul was a strong one. There were, of course, occasional arguments but with a strong commitment to our little family we always made up and life carried on as usual.

At this point I was working two nights a week, which were usually split so I didn't have to sleep all day the following day and could be with my children. Whilst on my nights off from work I didn't find out what had happened to the bat and to be honest I'd not given it a second thought.

Then during my next night shift I was leaving the nursery at around 2 a.m. when suddenly the bat appeared, swooping from the top of the big marble staircase. I screamed and Carla and I retreated quickly back through the nursery door.

She revealed that this had happened the night before and

she had instructed the staff working with her to open the enormous triple-bolted double doors at the entrance of the home and to turn the outside lights on and the inside lights off, in an attempt to lure the creature out.

'I thought it had left!' she exclaimed, as I peered ashen-faced through the glass panel to see if I could catch another glimpse. 'We saw it leave last night, so this must be another one!'

'Oh my goodness,' I thought, 'What if there is more than one?'

Carla recounted how the previous night one of my colleagues had seen the bat fly out of the door and had quickly dashed to close it, bolting the lock for good measure – as if it could open the door!

'Now you need to do the same,' she instructed. 'Go and open the doors, turn the lights on outside, then come back in here.'

'But I'm scared!' I pleaded. 'I'm really frightened of bats.'

Her face said it all and I knew that I didn't have any option to argue.

Quickly I left the safety of the nursery and ran to the door. I felt quite hysterical as I was convinced the bat could fly at me and get tangled in my hair. It was on a par with my fear of cockroaches – aarghh!

Typically the moment I switched off the lights one of the doors of the postnatal bedrooms opened to reveal a mother coming out to use the bathroom. She eyed me in a puzzled fashion, clearly wondering why I was stood in the dark with the house doors wide open.

'Is everything OK?' she asked.

'Yeah, everything is fine,' I trilled in my most reassuring voice. She didn't look convinced but relented and headed off to the loo. On her way back the situation remained unchanged except the doors were unguarded and Carla and I were hiding behind another door.

'Go and reassure that lady,' Carla commanded. So, petrified, I left the nursery once more to see if the mother was OK.

'Do you need anything?' I asked quietly, trying not to let her hear the tremble in my voice.

'No, I am fine,' she answered, eyeing me suspiciously. 'Are you expecting someone?'

'No,' I replied, 'it's just getting a bit warm in here.' It wasn't a convincing answer but she seemed to accept it and went back to bed. Phew! I ran back to safety.

After thirty minutes of us staring through the glass at the staircase and foyer area searching for signs of our unwanted guest, Carla told me to switch the lights back on.

'I think it must have left,' she concluded, so I did as instructed. We didn't see the bat again that night or indeed for the next week.

Then, two weeks later, at the start of my shift, I was doing my usual rounds checking on the mothers and babies and making sure they had enough supplies of nappies and cotton wool, when I had to go into the 'bat room' as it was now firmly ingrained in my mind, to check on a new mum and her tiny charge.

'Is there anything you need?' I asked the woman who was sat in a big chair breastfeeding her baby. She had her legs and feet tucked under her chair.

'Actually, I'm not sure how many nappies I have,' she said. 'Would you mind checking for me?'

As I bent down to look in the cupboard I suddenly saw a flash of black from under her chair.

'Aargh, it's a bat!' I shrieked.

'A rat?' the woman exclaimed, springing out of her seat and trying to get on the bed with her baby. As she did there was another flash of black and I noticed with dismay that she wearing black slippers. Oops.

'Oh,' I said. 'No, it's nothing. I just thought there was something on your slipper.'

As I laughed nervously and with embarrassment, she eyed me like I was going mad. Composing myself I sat on the bed.

'I am so sorry if I startled you,' I told her. Then I sat with her for a while until she seemed calm again.

I never did see that blasted bat again but for a long time I was on edge. It really gave me, and many other members of staff, the creeps!

However, it wasn't the only time we got spooked at Bramley Meade. One frosty night at around 10 p.m. one of my midwife colleagues, Tina, came running into the staff sitting room in a terrible state.

She reported that she'd been in the milk kitchen washing up the plastic boxes we filled with sterilising solution when she'd seen two men lurking on the fire escape, outside the window on the next level up. Her blood ran cold and she ran out of the room to alert us to call the police.

Thankfully the police arrived quickly and caught the men red-handed. Only it wasn't at all what it seemed. It turned out the men were from the council and had arrived to grit the fire escape. But instead of telling anyone, they'd just got on with the job in hand, which was a bit silly seeing as it was such a very remote place.

When it came to our nightly workload we seemed to either be desperately quiet or rushed off our feet and there were certainly a fair few hair-raising moments at Bramley Meade when everything seemed to happen at once.

I can remember one night when I was the only midwife working and I found myself caring for three women in labour during my twelve-hour shift. I was working alongside a helpful auxiliary nurse but she couldn't provide midwifery care. It was a hard night's work, though luckily there were actually only two women in labour at any one time.

It started with two women who had both been admitted that night at the same stage of labour. The birth rooms, or labour rooms as they were called then, were opposite each other and I was rushing from one room to the next, praying that both women wouldn't reach the point of actually giving birth at the same time. Both women and their partners knew about each other as I had to keep leaving each room to check on the other couple. As I dashed from one room to another I did my best to assure them that I was always close by.

I'd also informed the staff at Queens Park of the situation. It was important that they knew in case I needed them to send help. At one stage I thought that was going to be necessary as both women were progressing quickly and seemingly in tandem. But then one of the women started to push and her baby was born within minutes. Happy that all was well I left her and her husband to get acquainted with their new tiny tot and then dashed over the corridor to assist with the second birth.

Afterwards I saw the proud new fathers smiling broadly and having a great chat with each other about their new arrivals, which was very touching.

I'd just breathed a sigh of relief and started to relax when the phone went. 'Hello,' said the voice, 'My wife is having contractions every three minutes. I need to bring her in . . .'

Of course while these women had to share my time, at least there were separate labour rooms for each of them. My sister Anne, who had worked as a staff nurse at Bramley Meade for ten years before I started there, once told me about a time when two women would give birth in the same room.

This was when Bramley Meade was at its busiest time and there were many more births there. Anne recalled how the labour beds were separated by no more than a mobile screen.

'There were often two women in labour at once and each woman could hear exactly what was going on with the other,' Anne revealed.

She also remembered occasions when the midwife would dash from woman to woman with babies being born literally minutes apart in the same room.

The midwife would deliver one baby, quickly wash her hands and change her gloves, then go round the screen to deliver the next. Then, after more handwashing and glove changes, she would go back and forth delivering each placenta. Anne described it as being fairly stressful for her, but that the midwife seemed to take it in her stride and was very calm.

On one of my busier days I can remember receiving a call from a frantic husband to say he was bringing his wife in as she was in labour. Within minutes his car screeched up at the front door. Hearing the banging on the door and the bell being pressed frantically we rushed to the entrance to find his wife literally about to drop in the car. It was dark and cold and the car was cramped to say the least. The woman had slid down the front seat and in her fear was screaming at us to help her.

'Try not to push,' we encouraged her, 'Can you make it inside?'

Calmly but swiftly we supported her into the building and to her (and our!) relief we managed to get her inside into one of the empty postnatal rooms just as the baby's head began to appear. Within minutes, there were smiles and tears of joy as her baby was born safe and well.

But often time wouldn't be on our side, and babies would be born in an ambulance en route, on the road, in the grounds of Bramley Meade, or in one case just in the doorway!

It was my friend and colleague Pam who recounted this story of the time a labouring woman had come to Bramley Meade one morning with her husband. Whilst her husband was parking she announced at the door that her baby was 'coming out'.

She was wearing a shalwar kameez, which consists of a loose-fitting dress top and baggy trousers. To Pam's utter astonishment, when she went to examine the woman she discovered the baby nestling inside the trousers, having already been born! She quickly got help and took the mother and baby to a nearby room where they were given attention and congratulations.

Another member of staff, Julie, revealed how when she was in labour with her own third child her husband had sped down the bypass to Whalley as she felt like her baby was coming imminently. As she arrived at the front door an ambulance was arriving too at great speed and as it swerved to avoid their car it drove straight across the huge flowerbed that formed a small roundabout at the front of the home.

As my friend Julie was struggling out of her car with contractions coming thick and fast, the ambulance man was quickly ushering the other woman across the rose bushes into the building, in a similar state of urgency.

Both women were immediately taken off to have their babies and Julie's embarrassed husband then set to work helping the ambulance to reverse off the flowerbed.

Like Julie I too was to have my next baby at Bramley Meade.

I'd always wanted more children so in 1983 Paul and I were delighted to discover we were expecting again. We hadn't been trying or preventing; I was still only twenty-eight and we were just letting things happen. I went to the GP for a test and he confirmed the pregnancy.

We were thrilled and, apart from the usual morning sickness, at the start everything seemed to be going smoothly. Then in July 1983, when I was seven months' pregnant, my eldest sister Lynne went into a local private hospital to have a routine hysterectomy.

Lynne, who worked at the hospital where she'd have the operation, had experienced problems for a while and told us she was opting for the surgery as she felt, in her experience, that younger women tended to get over the procedure much faster.

The operation went according to plan and Chris, Lynne's husband, reported back that she was doing well. The hospital rules restricted visitors for the first two days after surgery and although Mum really wanted to see Lynne she had to wait, sending flowers instead.

Two days after Lynne's operation, on the Sunday, it was a beautiful sunny day so Paul and I took Anna and James to the seaside for a picnic. We had a great time and were still chatting and laughing as we arrived home.

As we were unpacking the car, one of our friends, Alex, was driving past the house when he stopped and called Paul over just as I was bundling the children through the front door.

While Paul was chatting I took Anna and James upstairs to get them ready for bed. I'd just got them in the bath when Paul came in and took hold of my hands. The look on his face scared me.

'What are you doing?' I said.

'Sheena,' he replied. 'Lynne died.'

For a minute I didn't understand.

'What do you mean?' I asked. As Paul started to cry, the full horror of what I was hearing hit me. Paul explained that Alex, who was also friends with Lynne, had heard that she'd passed away that day. She'd been killed instantly by a blood clot from the surgery. When Alex had seen us unloading the car with big smiles on our faces he knew that we hadn't heard.

'No, it can't be true!' I cried, my voice shaking. Then I ran from the bathroom leaving my family. I was heavily pregnant and almost fell downstairs but my first thought was my mum and Lynne's children.

I picked up the phone and tried to dial Mum's number but my hands were shaking. Dropping the receiver, I started to cry. Paul couldn't come to me as the children were in the bath.

As I sobbed all different thoughts were swimming around my head. It was my worst nightmare. How could someone so close to me and so young at forty, far too young, die like this, just out of the blue? I couldn't think straight.

Then the phone rang. It was Anne, my next eldest sister, the strong one who always seems to pull us together in times of trouble.

'Come over to my house,' she instructed me. Putting the receiver down I ran around the house in a complete haze, looking for my keys and bag, and then within minutes I was in the car driving down the road to my sister's house.

My heart was pounding in my chest and my throat felt tight. I still couldn't believe it and could hardly see where I was going as the tears poured down my face.

I was to learn more horrendous details when I found Mum at Anne's, incredibly composed but totally shattered with grief. Even though Mum knew she wasn't allowed to visit Lynne, she had been out with her friend Sylvia that morning and as she was passing the hospital anyway, decided spontaneously to pop in.

Walking in, Mum and her friend didn't see any staff members so they headed straight to Room Ten, which they knew was Lynne's room as Mum had sent the flowers there.

When Mum walked in she was shocked to see a body laid out and wrapped in a sheet. Confused but aware of what she was seeing due to her experience working in a hospital, Mum looked round the room and spotted the flowers she'd sent the previous day. Presuming Lynne had been temporarily moved to another room she went out again to look for her and was greeted by a member of staff in the corridor.

She introduced herself as Lynne Simm's mother and asked why there was a dead body in her daughter's room. With colour draining from her cheeks, the nurse ushered my mother and her friend into a nearby office.

It was at that moment that Mum knew there was something dreadfully wrong.

After the terrible news was broken to her she discovered that Chris had been nearby when Lynne had collapsed and was in the building whilst attempts were being made to resuscitate her.

Distraught and helpless, Chris had headed home to find Cathy, his teenage daughter, and to call his other daughter, Paula, who was married with children of her own and lived in London. It was then he realised my mum wasn't home. He'd called my sisters who eventually tracked Mum down. The whole family was devastated and stunned. We grouped together and our attention revolved round Chris, Paula, Cathy and Mum.

Mum was incredibly brave, and almost warrior-like as

she tried to support everyone else, but she never really recovered from Lynne's death. She was truly broken-hearted and the hardest period must have come after her stroke three years later when she was unable to tell us how sad she was.

Cathy spent time with Mum, and they became incredibly close. They supported and helped each other in the healing process – both had a gap that was impossible to fill.

I had been pregnant when my dad died, and here I was again in this dreadful fog, trying hard not to crumble. I was so very sad, and at the funeral I cried so much that I worried my growing unborn baby may be affected.

Two months later I went into labour.

Thankfully I'd just spent a very pleasant and cathartic two-week break in Cornwall with Paul, Anna and James. The time away had left me feeling properly rested and happy for really the first time since Lynne's death.

I'd asked Carla Gazzola, by this time my close friend as well as my colleague, to be my midwife, and when my contractions came first thing in the morning Paul took me to Bramley Meade, leaving the children with Mum.

It was surreal being driven to my workplace knowing that this time I would be the one being cared for rather than the other way round. As it happened I would be absolutely delighted with the experience and would get to see first-hand how fabulous the midwifery care was from the other side.

Again my labour was hard and just as painful but also very straightforward and productive. I felt comfortable and easy in this homely environment with no hustle and bustle at all. Carla was the most wonderful midwife to me. She was gentle and calm and her approach really worked with my plan for Tom's birth. I had asked her not to put her hands on my abdomen or examine me too much and she followed my wishes to the letter. She also said very little. Carla's midwifery skills, manner and approach were ones that I tried to emulate over the years.

For the first time I tried a visualisation technique that I'd been told about by some of the mothers who had undergone National Childbirth Trust (NCT) antenatal sessions before their births. I had also seen this technique work in practice.

'You need to practise thinking about a calming image,' they explained. 'Then when your contraction comes you need to focus on it in your mind.'

My 'picture' was a beautiful island and I was in a boat. When the contraction came I imagined myself rowing to the island, ebbing back and forth in the water as the waves of contraction hit me. When the contraction was at its peak and most painful I imagined I was halfway there. As it faded away, I imagined reaching the island. It really worked for me and I was calm and relaxed all the way through. In fact Carla said she could only tell I was going through a contraction by listening to my breathing.

She obviously knew all about what had happened to Lynne just a few months beforehand so she was very caring towards all my family as well.

When I was in advanced labour Carla whispered in my ear that Mum had arrived, with her friend Sylvia, to see me, and that she wanted to come in to be with me for the birth. I agreed immediately as Mum was still desperately sad and I thought it would be something positive for her to focus on. I invited Sylvia to come in too as I knew she hadn't had any children of her own and had never seen a baby born. Although I was concentrating hard I opened my eyes and looked into Mum's for a moment to let her know I was very happy to have her there.

I closed my eyes again and with a final push my baby was born easily and lifted into my arms. A beautiful bald little baby boy! We marvelled at how Thomas, as we called him, was so strikingly different from Anna and James, who'd both been born with an abundance of black hair.

Paul and I loved him instantly and couldn't stop admiring him and showering him with kisses and cuddles before he was passed around to be admired by all the family. I felt much more alert after the birth this time round and felt like I was glowing with happiness.

Anna and James came to see me shortly afterwards and were totally thrilled and excited about their new brother.

We also asked Carla to be one of Tom's godmothers, and to our delight she accepted. After that she always had a special bond with Tom; she just loved him and for years to come they would spend hours and hours together. What an extraordinary midwife Carla was. I will never forget how she cared for me.

Mum loved the experience and talked about it for ages afterwards. When I went home she spent lots of time with me, keeping busy and helping me, which I appreciated more than she ever knew.

Chapter 8

'You're almost there!' I said, urging the mother, who was clearly using every last bit of energy to give the final push that would bring her baby into the world.

Her face contorted with concentration as she gave a last heave, she pushed out her baby into my waiting hands. He lay there blinking as he took in the world for the very first time.

Glancing at the clock I made a note of the time. Three minutes past midnight.

'Your Christmas baby is here!' I smiled. 'Congratulations!'

Earlier that evening I'd arrived to work my Christmas Eve shift. After a busy day preparing the turkey and vegetables and wrapping the children's presents I'd left home, leaving Paul on Santa duties.

I often worked over the festive period, either doing a Christmas Eve shift (and rushing home to my children on Christmas morning) or covering Christmas night.

If my shift dictated that I came home on Christmas morning, Paul would wait with the children until I arrived then they'd be allowed to go downstairs to see what Santa had brought. This was particularly hard for the children who were beside themselves with anticipation, but also hard for Paul. Overnight he'd have to sort out the stockings full of presents, drink Santa's milk, scoff the mince pies and attend to excitable children determined not to sleep – all by himself. No easy feat!

As I walked through the main entrance I was reminded of the wonders of the festive season, the smell of the pine tree, the decorations and the lights.

Christmases were particularly special at Bramley as our lovely, cosy maternity unit was as close to being at home as you could possibly get in an NHS institution. Every year, decorations were carefully positioned throughout the building by the staff and the hall was filled with the sound of carols and Christmas tunes. Smells of home cooking wafted from the kitchen and there was a lovely snug, jolly feeling about the place as the festive season drew near.

On that cold Christmas Eve in 1984, the home had a calm, quiet atmosphere as most of the mothers and babies had gone home for the festive celebrations.

As I crossed the hall and strolled along the corridor to find Carla I'd wondered if overnight we'd have a special Christmas baby.

When I found Carla she reported that there was indeed a woman in labour. But seeing as the labour was progressing well she suspected the baby would be born before 25 December arrived.

It was just after 9 p.m. that I headed into the dimly lit labour room to meet Sandra, who was in labour with her third baby. Her husband Tony was supporting her well as she breathed in the gas and air with each strong contraction.

For the next couple of hours Sandra concentrated hard and dozed between contractions while I held whispered conversations with Tony to support him.

Then as midnight approached, things began to speed up. By 11.55 p.m. I could see the baby's head. Eight minutes later baby James arrived – a perfect Christmas baby, healthy and strong.

Christmas babies at Bramley Meade were considered very special and as was tradition James was placed in a beautifully decorated cot and received gifts of a teddy bear and bootees. Sandra's present was some toiletries for her to pamper herself with in the forthcoming days although of course the best gift she could ever imagine was nestling in her arms already.

Another tradition at Bramley was to order a huge Christmas tree that would stand outside the house. I can remember one year when one of my colleagues, Kerry, asked the caretaker, whose job it was to order in the impressive festive centrepiece, if she could order a tree for herself too. The order was made and a few weeks later the trees arrived.

But Kerry was perplexed by the size of her tree; it was larger than she'd expected so when her husband came to collect her that evening after work they duly hacked off the bottom and heaved it on to the roof of their car, securing it with straps to get it home. Unfortunately what Kerry didn't realise was that she'd actually butchered the massive tree that was supposed to adorn the entrance of Bramley Meade.

As she'd driven her huge tree home, a small household-sized one was sitting unloved in the corner of the foyer. By the time Kerry's mistake was realised it was too late to order a new tree so for that Christmas we had to make do with the poxy little one that was pretty much swamped by the impressive frontage of Bramley Meade.

Poor Kerry. She was justifiably mortified and for the rest of her time at Bramley suffered much teasing from the other staff over her festive faux pas.

Not that she was the only one to come a Christmas cropper . . .

On a yearly basis local carol singers, loved by both the mothers and staff, would arrive to sing. However, one Christmas they were inadvertently sent packing by my flummoxed friend Elaine.

Elaine was busy caring for a woman in labour when she heard the front doorbell ringing. When it carried on and no one answered, Elaine rushed downstairs to see what all the fuss was about.

'Carol singers!' a jolly man standing on the doorstep said.

'Sorry, but there is no one here with that name,' Elaine retorted, promptly closing the door. The singers, probably very perplexed, then left the grounds and Elaine quickly returned to her responsibilities without giving it a second thought.

It was only later when another member of staff commented that it was odd the singers hadn't turned up that the penny dropped. As she admitted her mistake the laughter could be heard throughout the building and the smiles over that particular story continued for decades.

With doctors largely involved in the ongoing care of the women we saw at Bramley Meade it was not unusual to have a family GP arrive at all times of the day or night to be there for a patient as she gave birth.

We kept the doctors' phone numbers in a small book in the staff office and if they'd requested to be present we'd call them when the woman was ready to push. Some of the GPs were very hands-on, dashing into the building raring to help. Others would sit outside so as not to interfere but would be around in case a problem occurred.

On the whole we had very good relationships with the local doctors and I always felt there was a certain amount of mutual trust between the two professions. But we midwives also felt that having another person in the room just at the most sensitive and crucial time changed the atmosphere and could be off-putting for women.

Another concern for us was the way some more interfering GPs pulled rank with unwanted instructions at the last minute. Dr Blare was one such GP that we dreaded calling. This doctor was of the 'old school' and had done his obstetric (maternity) training in the years of routine episiotomy – the procedure I had originally seen at the first birth I witnessed as a pupil midwife.

He believed that all women having their first baby should have their perineum cut with scissors to help the head come through. Often he'd walk into the room completely clueless as to how the birth was proceeding and would not hesitate in calling out, 'Do an episiotomy, Sister!' (He always called every midwife Sister.)

So after a while we developed an unspoken strategy to call Dr Blare, and some other doctors, only when it was almost too late and the woman was already pushing. Dr

Blare would jump in his car and hurtle down the road to Bramley but more often than not by the time he arrived the baby was already born and the women would be saved from enduring the unnecessary procedure.

Of course, most of the GPs were lovely and the women were delighted to see them and show off their new babies. Plus there were times when we really needed the skills of the GPs – perhaps if a woman needed stitches that were beyond our capabilities.

One of my favourite GPs was Dr Ainsworth from Whalley. Everyone loved him. He was humble and pleasant and always keen to help.

'If you are worried, call me, even if I am not on call,' he'd say. 'I'll be with you in a jiffy!'

One night during a difficult birth I called him at home, apologising for waking him.

'Not a problem,' he told me. 'I'm on my way.'

True to his word, he pulled up outside ten minutes later and when he dashed into the building I was both amused and impressed to see he was still wearing his pyjamas.

After scrubbing up and donning a surgical gown he rushed in to help his very grateful patient give birth to a beautiful baby girl.

I am pleased to report, though, that in the eight years I worked at Bramley Meade I didn't see one serious incident during labour, and when emergencies did happen they were rare. We had no doctors on site and apart from the odd bit of tricky stitching we didn't need them.

If a labour was delayed or taking too long and I felt the woman needed extra assistance I would sometimes call

Queens Park and arrange an ambulance transfer. On these rare occasions, if staffing levels permitted, one of us would go with her to the hospital so the woman didn't have the stress of changing midwives.

One evening at around 10 p.m. a woman called Ruth came into Bramley Meade, having called us to say her contractions were coming regularly.

When she arrived with David, her partner, her contractions were strong, and she started using gas and air straight away. Ruth was five centimetres dilated when I examined her – your cervix needs to be ten centimetres dilated before your body is ready to give birth – and the baby, her first, was doing fine.

Ruth's labour progressed well until she was eight centimetres dilated but then although her contractions continued to be regular and strong there was no further dilatation. When I examined her at midnight, four hours later, there was still no change.

The baby's position was posterior (the baby's back to the mother's back) and I had been keeping Ruth mobile to encourage the baby to move.

I called the midwife in charge of the labour ward at Queens Park and explained Ruth's situation. We agreed that because there were no other problems we would wait to see how things were at the next check-up.

But when I went back into the room Ruth's waters had broken and there was meconium in the fluid (a sign the baby had had its bowels open and could be distressed).

Although the baby's heartbeat was still good I now thought Ruth could need further assistance.

'I think it would be better if you went to the hospital now, Ruth,' I explained. 'Your baby may be a little distressed but we have time and will look after you.'

Ruth, now panting heavily and in the midst of her contractions, nodded.

I organised the ambulance and after about thirty-five minutes Ruth was on her way.

There were three of us midwives on that night so I was able to go with her in the ambulance while David followed in his car.

When Ruth was examined on the labour ward she was still eight centimetres but eventually managed to give birth to a baby boy with help from the ventouse machine – where a small suction cap is applied to the baby's head to gently move it down the birth canal. Then it was celebrations all round as Ruth and David cuddled up to their new son, Joseph.

On another occasion my colleague Sandra was caring for a woman in labour and as time went by she did a vaginal examination to see how things were progressing. Sandra felt the baby's cord pulsating in front of the baby's head and was concerned that as the head came down the birth canal the blood supply to the baby could be cut off.

Following procedure, Sandra kept her fingers inside the woman's vagina to keep the baby's head off the cord. Meanwhile the hospital was alerted and an emergency ambulance called. Sandra had to keep the pressure off throughout the transfer to hospital and indeed up to the point the woman went into the operating theatre for a Caesarean section. Mother and baby were both well and Sandra says it was one birth she will never forget.

A happy ending all round but it served as a reminder to us midwives that the unexpected can happen during childbirth and that we must have the appropriate skills to deal with emergencies and to refer on to doctors when necessary.

Sadly I can recall one tragedy in the early years I worked at Bramley Meade but the outcome would not have been any different if the woman had been in a hospital where doctors were.

It was as one of my midwife colleagues was feeding the babies in the nursery that they noticed that one was not breathing. It was an enormous shock, and although resuscitation was attempted the baby died. The midwife who found the baby was inconsolable and the parents completely distraught.

Investigations revealed no abnormality, so cot death was given as a verdict. It took a long time for the staff to recover from such an event.

As my working years flew by at Bramley Meade my little family also grew.

Anna and James were proving to be very theatrical, entertaining us on a nightly basis with Anna's dancing and James's acting. His favourite character was Fagin from *Oliver!* and he frequently had us in stitches impersonating him. On one occasion a neighbour reported that James was sat on a branch of a tree that overhung the main road singing, 'If I Were a Rich Man!' from *Fiddler on the Roof* at the top of his voice. She was horrified.

Tom was gentle, good at football and a pleasure to have around. He loved dressing up as Superman and 'flying' around the bedroom. They were lovely children and we had lots of fun as they grew up.

The children always had loads of friends running around the garden and we used to sledge in the winter and picnic in summer. And of course dear Carla used to come over on her nights off to cook and help me.

In the three years since my sister Lynne's death Mum had done her best to stay upbeat, as we all had, but there was no doubt she felt a deep loss and sadness every day.

Touchingly she also formed a firm bond with Cathy, Lynne's daughter, who she saw regularly. One day in 1986, Cathy, by now training to be a nurse in London, had come up north for the weekend and she and Mum went shopping to find a new dress for Christmas.

As they travelled into town together on the bus Mum bumped her head on the stairs but seemed OK. But later back home, when Mum went upstairs to try her new dress on, Cathy heard her making a funny noise.

When she investigated, Mum wasn't able to speak coherently so she called the local doctor.

The doctor arrived but when Mum's speech returned he said he was happy with her condition and left. That night Eileen stayed over at Mum's and was able to talk to her about what happened. Mum explained what a terrible experience it was when she wasn't able to make herself understood. What we didn't know was that she'd go on to endure this for the next twenty-four years.

Mum had suffered a stroke and in the night must have had a further bleed in her brain. By the morning she had completely lost her speech and her right side was weak, so she was admitted to hospital where she deteriorated rapidly.

Her condition was critical and she was unconscious for several days. There were times when we thought she wouldn't survive and each one of us was in the depths of despair again.

Mum was only sixty-three and had endured so many major illnesses in her life – not just her heart attack but also a hysterectomy – yet she always bounced back and became the strongest of us all. We wondered whether her luck had run out and if we were going to lose her.

For a terrible couple of nights we took it in turns spending hours slumped on chairs beside her bed, praying that she'd pull through.

Days later, after pacing up and down the corridors and shedding oceans of tears, Mum started to improve.

We never left her alone when she was in hospital, and this was to become a normal pattern in years to come when she lost her ability to speak. Every time she was admitted to hospital we stayed with her without fail.

However, as Mum slowly gained strength, it became apparent that she had lost the use of her right side and her speech had completely gone. Sounds came out jumbled, apart from a few words that we learned to know and love over the years.

Mum eventually came home and stayed with my sister Anne.

With Mum now needing constant care I was very touched as Carla sprung into action, supporting me at work and at home. The truth is that, without her, I would have been stuck, and the thought did cross my mind that I might have to give up work.

But Carla would arrive to help make meals for my family or to just sit and listen as I cried. She was great with the children, always ready with a little game or activity to keep them entertained. She stepped into Mum's shoes in many ways and became like a grandma to Anna, James and Tom.

When she babysat for us I'd come home to discover she'd done my ironing, cooked a mouthwatering dish for dinner or knitted something for one of the kids.

She also used to invite the children to Bramley Meade to play and subsequently they all have lovely memories of seeing newborn babies and playing in the grounds.

While juggling my home and work life was as hard as ever, now I was an experienced midwife I was constantly reminded why I loved my job so much.

It wasn't just about 'delivering babies', it was building relationships and trust that I cherished. It was wonderful when couples specifically asked for me to deliver their babies because friends had recommended me. I was also chuffed when mothers requested me when they came back a second or third time.

I loved making new friends and sharing couples' joyful moments. There was a lot of time for that at Bramley Meade, which I really enjoyed.

However, when occasionally I'd get asked to help with staffing shortages at Queens Park Hospital, it was a very different environment. Not only was it much busier, but amusingly the midwives at Queens Park seemed to view

Bramley Meade as some sort of hippy commune. And when I arrived with my plaited long hair and 'Jesus sandals' I'm not sure I helped!

The dress code at Bramley was the same as in my early years as a nurse in Blackburn – nurses' uniform with a zip at the front and a starched collar and cap. But it was definitely more relaxed than at the hospital and many of us wore sandals for comfort on the night shift.

While no one batted an eyelid about my relaxed attire at Bramley, it was to cause a stir at Queens.

Bounding into the staffroom on one night I'd been called in I found a senior midwife.

'I've come to help!' I said.

'Oh,' she said, taking a good look. 'It's the farmyard midwife!' I noticed she was eyeing my feet.

'Those shoes!' she exclaimed. 'You look like a hippy!' All the other staff in the room looked at each other and smiled. Suddenly I realised how differently I was dressed from everyone else. Oops. Feeling slightly embarrassed I sloped off to the labour ward to see what I could do.

The labour ward was very busy and I felt nervous and less confident. The women having their babies at Queens Park were more likely to have complications and the whole atmosphere seemed fraught.

Naturally it took me longer to do everything as I didn't know where things were. I felt like I was being slow even though the midwives I was working with were lovely and seemed appreciative of an extra pair of hands.

I'd return to Bramley Meade feeling satisfied that I'd helped but also relieved to be back. But what I didn't realise was that my days there were numbered. Over the next few years, more and more women would be having their babies at Queens Park while the number of deliveries at Bramley Meade would start to dwindle.

While for many years Bramley had been thriving, gradually the number of women being booked in by GPs diminished. This was largely to do with changes in the way GPs worked 'on call'.

Previously doctors were on call for their own patients, but a new system evolved where GPs in a geographical area would now take it in turns to cover their patch and consequently a wider spectrum of patients.

It meant that GPs wouldn't necessarily be available to attend at the birth if their patient went to Bramley. At the same time there seemed to be a shift in advice with many expectant mothers wrongly being told that it was 'safer' to have a baby in hospital.

At first we were confused by the dwindling numbers and couldn't understand why so many pregnancies were now being booked into Queens Park. But when we spoke to women at the antenatal clinics it all became clear.

There were other factors too. New guidance was introduced, restricting the number of women eligible for delivery at Bramley Meade. Now only women who had previously had normal births could go there. At the same time the women who used to come to us to convalesce after their birth were now being sent home to do so instead.

It made me sad, as I loved the ethos at Bramley Meade. Together my colleagues and I had learned how to be skilful midwives who didn't rely on unnecessary interventions such as electronic monitoring machines to assess mothers and babies who are at low risk.

Because women had the continuous support of one midwife, it was rare that she needed strong painkilling drugs such as pethidine. If she did request the drug, or if the midwife suggested it, we would usually give half a dose (50 mgs), and that always seemed to be enough. Often when women don't have support or the birth environment is wrong, the pain they feel during a contraction intensifies and more drugs are used. Before and after my experience at Bramley Meade, when I was working in hospital environments, women would sometimes have up to 300 mg of pethidine over several doses, which increases drowsiness and can have an effect on the baby's condition at birth. But most women didn't use any drugs at Bramley, apart from gas and air. We also encouraged women to use water to help ease their labour pain. We didn't have birth pools, but we'd run them a deep bath and they'd stay in there for hours.

Sometimes, in the wee small hours, I would sit with women who were breastfeeding their babies. We would chat about all kinds of things and sometimes women felt comfortable enough to tell me their little worries or concerns. I loved those times. It seemed very close and intimate and a great privilege for me to be in a position where I could listen and perhaps support women if they needed it.

Many bonds were made and even recently I met two women in Clitheroe who remembered me from Bramley Meade. They mentioned our little 'night chats' and how much they'd enjoyed them. It is a great feeling when women and their partners remember you.

*

The years passed and I continued to deliver babies and enjoy family life as my children grew into little characters. I loved watching them blossom but Paul and I still fancied adding to our brood. In 1989 we were blessed with another little Byrom baby. In August that year I was to go on maternity leave for a final time.

I'd actually had two miscarriages in between this pregnancy and giving birth to Tom so it was with some relief that I made it full-term.

I worked up until I was about thirty-four weeks' pregnant (in other words, six weeks before my due date), which was very tiring, but I got loads of help from Carla, who used to pop round just to 'be there', and also from my friends Pat and Jill.

Although I desperately wanted Carla to be my midwife again there was no guarantee she'd be available as it could have been her night off. But as luck would have it I felt my first twinge of labour while I was taking a stroll with her. It was the afternoon of her last day off before her stint of night shifts began and I knew she was about to work seven nights on the trot. If I progressed slowly throughout the day then she might just get to catch my baby.

Later that day, as I kept busy at home, my labour advanced steadily, so in the evening I called my friend Pat and asked her to come and mind the children. She arrived at 8 p.m. but I deliberately waited until 9 p.m. (the time Carla began her shift) before Paul and I set off to Bramley Meade.

Pat was as excited as we were and hugged me before I

left. As a strong contraction hit me I suddenly felt apprehensive. I suddenly realised how distinctive the pain was – in between babies I'd forgotten!

'What have I done?' I exclaimed to Pat.

'You'll be just fine,' she laughed.

In the car Paul and I talked excitedly about our new baby. What would it be? A boy or a girl? We had one girl and two boys already so we really wanted a sister for Anna.

Bramley Meade was only round the corner from where we lived, so within minutes we were arriving, to be greeted by Carla who was as calm and gentle as always.

As my contractions became more frequent and stronger I started to use the same visualisation strategy I'd used when in labour with Thomas and it helped very much again.

Carla supported me in her usual quiet way, remembering how I didn't like to be touched. She'd prepared the room with soft lighting and loads of cushions scattered around, and there was a birth mat ready and waiting if I wanted it. Like many of the other midwives at Bramley, Carla was a real advocate for promoting normal birth and encouraging women to be as active as possible in labour. But I felt tired and wanted to rest so I lay on my side and focused on that faraway island. This time the distinct urge to push came sooner than with my other children and our fourth little baby slithered into the world with ease. With a huge grin I lifted up my baby for the first time and marvelled at her – a little girl!

Paul was beside me planting kisses on our new baby's

cheeks and when I looked into his eyes I saw tears of joy. In that moment we felt so blessed to have four healthy children – two of each sex!

'It doesn't get better than this,' he whispered. At last our family was complete.

Our brilliant GP, Dr Alasdair Carter, who'd also attended Tom's birth, arrived just before Olivia was born but stayed outside the room. Afterwards we invited him in to meet our daughter and he drank chilled champagne with us all to celebrate.

Shortly afterwards, my sister Anne arrived and helped me to have a bath. As I lay back in the relaxing warm water we chatted about the miracle of having babies.

After the birth I was moved to a lovely upstairs single room that used to be home to an ex-senior midwife, Mrs Marsden. I can still remember the wonderful moment when James, Anna and Tom came running up the stairs to see me. They were so excited and had made cards with Pat that morning and drawn pictures for their new baby sister.

The room was grand and had an en-suite bathroom with an antique clawed bath. It also had a huge double-door antique wardrobe that housed the chocolates left for the staff from appreciative families. Every now and then the chocolates were taken out and divided amongst the staff. We used to get our quota in a piece of tissue or a paper towel. This arrangement was not a great one, as half the chocolates would have gone off and would have a white film over them by the time we got them. Ugh.

Lying in bed looking at the wardrobe made me giggle, as

I remembered one night when my midwife friend Tina and I happened to be working together and the need for chocolate became too much.

As Tina and I were both part-time midwives we usually worked a shift with one of the sisters. But not that night, as they were on holiday. It was the perfect moment to launch 'Operation Chocolate Storm'.

It all began with me whining to Tina that I was hungry.

'I could just eat some chocolate right now,' I said. As I looked at her I could see that the same evil thought had sprung to her mind too. We could raid the wardrobe!

The wardrobe was locked and the key was kept in the manager's desk but after rummaging through we were disappointed not to find it.

By this stage we were so fixated with the thought of chocolate that we crept up the main staircase and checked out the lock on the wardrobe itself.

'It's no good,' Tina exclaimed. 'The doors are locked and very secure.'

But then we noticed that if we pulled hard enough the doors parted slightly, and the lock became dislodged. So we started pulling until eventually one door flew open and – oops – out popped a mountain of goodies!

For the next ten minutes we sat on the bed giggling and stuffing our faces with English and Belgian chocolates – that is, until gluttony and guilt set in and we both felt violently sick. Not our finest hour but we did enjoy it.

We made sure we closed the wardrobe doors carefully to cover our tracks and disposed of the boxes. Luckily for us no one ever discovered our secret, but Tina and I always used to giggle at the memory when chocolate allocation time came round again.

During my six-month maternity leave the number of women coming to Bramley Meade declined further. It was a sad time.

In its busiest era I would come to work at Bramley and care for twenty women who had given birth. Now the other midwives reported that sometimes there were only two or three.

Staff were being transferred to the hospital to work as it was busier there and, not surprisingly, discussions were being had as to the efficiency of the service. It was clear there were too many staff on each shift to care for so few women. I knew that Mrs Quinn, now head of midwifery and managing the whole of the maternity services in the area, was discussing the options carefully with her management team.

She felt there was inequality in the services women were receiving. It was very busy at Queens Park with not enough midwives and yet quiet at Bramley Meade with staff falling over themselves. By closing Bramley and transferring the staff to Queens Park Pauline also believed she could help to influence the philosophy of care at the hospital. By taking our skills there she hoped to promote the natural birth practices we'd developed over the years.

Consultations with the public took place and there was understandably quite a lot of resistance from local mothers and councillors but eventually a decision was made. I'd just returned from my maternity leave when it was announced that Bramley Meade was going to close.

Finally the sad day arrived and in 1990 I drove to Bramley Meade for the last time, my mind firmly fixed on that night nine years earlier when I'd left my two little ones at home and first driven to Whalley to start work. So much had happened since then and I had learned so much. I'd grown attached to Bramley and it seemed so sad to be leaving it.

In the weeks beforehand I knew my colleagues were feeling despondent too. Not only were we leaving each other but we were also leaving behind a beautiful building and a special period of our lives. There were very mixed feelings about the decision: some thought it was inevitable given the situation, others were angry and could not rationalise why the decision had been made. There had been much publicity in the press, but the bottom line was that the unit couldn't be sustained and Queens Park and the women using it needed us.

On my final shift there were no women in the home. It was just Kerry, an auxiliary nurse, and myself, there to keep watch on the very last day as there were still drugs on the premises that hadn't been removed.

As I walked around, nostalgically recalling all the babies and all the joy I'd witnessed within these walls, the silence was eerie. Thankfully Kerry, who loved telling stories, kept me occupied.

Looking back, Bramley Meade had been a fabulous place to work. Many of my midwifery colleagues who worked there in the 1980s agree that it was their best years. It was so homely and nurturing, the staff cared for each other, and we in turn cared for the women and facilitated birth with empathy and kindness.

I'd worked with some wonderful people but it was without a doubt Carla I was going to miss the most. Not only was she my midwife for the births of two of my children but she had also become a very close friend of my family. Carla had retired before Bramley Meade closed but as she lived in the building she stayed until the home finally closed its doors.

At that point she decided to move back to Italy to be near her family. Her departure was incredibly emotional. Carla had made so many friends and gained respect from colleagues and mothers alike. For her retirement we arranged a party for her and invited people from far and wide.

My son Thomas presented her with a small bouquet and my sister Eileen made her a fabulous cake. The biggest surprise for her was the entrance of a young man who she had cared for thirty-five years earlier when she'd first arrived in the UK to work as a nanny for a family in Manchester. We had tracked him down and secretly planned the reunion.

Today Carla still lives in Italy and we are in touch. I will never forget what she did for me and my family. Not only did she have an amazing influence on my career, she also has such a special place in my children's hearts.

Chapter 9

Walking swiftly through the department to fetch a drink for a labouring mum-to-be, Paula, I dodged out the way of a woman walking on to the labour ward clutching her swollen abdomen. She stopped to lean on a bar on the wall, breathing through her contraction.

The phone was ringing and Julie, one of the other midwives, rushed to answer it. A bell from one of the side rooms rang and seeing as there were no other midwives around, I went through the labour room door to answer the call.

There I found Rabia pushing and panting. 'Baby coming!' her husband said in broken English.

Rabia's midwife was out of the room, and her labour was obviously progressing quicker than expected. 'Welcome to Queens Park!' I thought.

To be honest the last place I'd expected to end up in was the labour ward. Prior to Bramley Meade closing all staff had been invited to meetings with Mrs Quinn and another manager who asked where we wanted to work once we were transferred to Queens Park.

I said that I didn't mind, as long as it wasn't the labour

ward. I felt my skills in caring for women with complications needed a brush-up. So of course that is exactly where I ended up!

Prior to my first shift I went to visit the ward, meet the staff and to discuss my night shifts. I had a contract to work night duty and I wanted to figure out how things would work in my new job.

The manager, Miss Davies, intimidated me from the first time I met her. She was medium height but slim, and in all the years I knew her I never once saw her smile. I always think it's very unnerving when you smile at someone and they look back at you stony-faced. I found her very stern.

'You won't be working nights,' she told me. 'We need you on days.'

I was very shocked to hear this as I had a contractual agreement that I'd be doing nights. Although I was happy to do day duties eventually, at this point I still had my small baby, Olivia, and working night duty meant I didn't have to rely on childcare as much. Paul was now working as a financial advisor for the Prudential and his working hours were sporadic.

But when I carefully tried to explain my personal situation Miss Davies was having none of it. Not only was I to work during the day, but my twenty-hour contract was going to be utilised by doing four five-hour shifts a week.

As she told me this I panicked about the repercussions on my family life and felt tears pricking in my eyes. How could I do that? It was impossible. I later learned that the management team had made a decision to try to swap day and night staff to ensure our skills were kept up-to-date, which makes sense – but at the time I left feeling totally miserable. I absolutely loved my job as a midwife but I was worried about leaving Olivia four days out of seven. The shift timings were difficult – the early shift started at 7.30 a.m. and the late shift finished at 9 p.m. – so my time with my other children would suffer too. We lived eight miles from the hospital so there would be travel time to take into account too. I had no idea who I could ask to look after them. Mum wasn't able to help now and Paul's mum wasn't around much.

As I drove home, the only solution seemed to be that I would have to leave. I was in floods of tears by the time I got home and immediately scooped Olivia up in my arms.

'Come on, She,' Paul said as I tearfully explained my predicament. 'Let's talk it through and see if we can find a solution.'

So we agreed that I would try to work the new shift patterns to see how it went. Thankfully we had brilliant friends and family who agreed to help us.

So overnight my job completely changed and I was plummeted into the working world of a high-risk maternity unit that was three times as busy as what I'd been used to.

My first morning was a total shock. Determined to make the most of my situation, I arrived for work bright-eyed and bushy-tailed.

The first task of the day was to attend a handover meeting where everyone was informed about the women in labour. As I stood there with my new colleagues I couldn't help feeling nervous. I wasn't a completely new face as they had seen me from time to time but I definitely felt like the new girl.

One told me later that she could not believe the way I was dressed. I'd arrived for work in my Jesus sandals as usual, with my long hair up in a bun. She said she thought I looked naïve. The Jesus sandals soon disappeared. I already felt like a fish out of water and they weren't helping.

After the meeting I was allocated a woman to care for – but also faced my first dilemma. The woman needed to be 'monitored' with an electronic cardiotocograph machine, which recorded the heartbeat of the baby and the mother's contractions. The straps of the machine were placed around her abdomen to hold small round plates (transducers) against the place where the heartbeat could be picked up.

I had limited experience with electronic cardiotocograph machines – we hadn't had them at Bramley, but I'd occasionally used one at Burnley many years previously. Now, faced with a pile of straps and plates, I couldn't quite remember what to do. Introducing myself to the woman and her partner I explained to them what the monitor did then I did my best to fit it.

But after several attempts to figure out why the machine wasn't picking up the heartbeat I was left with no choice but to slip out, red-faced, to find the shift leader and ask for help. Luckily the reaction I got was OK and I soon learned who my allies were and who would help me without retribution or comment.

One of my most-loved colleagues was a wonderful night sister called Katie Hindle. I first encountered Katie over the phone when she used to call up Bramley Meade every night at 12 p.m. to make sure everything was running smoothly. Whereas the other night sisters were very matter-of-fact, Katie always asked how you were.

'How are your children?' she'd trill. 'Are you well?' It was nice that she took such an interest in people and she always remembered details. When I moved to Queens Park I saw that she was like this with everyone. She was genuinely interested in other people and their lives. She was also obsessed with cleaning and was affectionately known on the wards as Sister J-Cloth as she always had one in her hand.

I'd never really considered myself as a 'career girl' but as I got to grips with daily life on the labour ward I continued to be passionate about midwifery and loved the part I played in women's lives during the birth of their baby.

With every birth I witnessed I felt grateful and privileged to work in such an extraordinary profession and the courage and strength of the labouring women never failed to amaze me.

I loved the companionship too: the other midwives and support workers were some of my dearest friends and we worked well together, supporting and encouraging each other during the busiest times.

But even though Bramley Meade and Queens Park Hospital Maternity Unit were part of the same Health Authority, that was where their similarities ended. The layout of the maternity unit was very hospital-orientated, with long Nightingale wards and very few side rooms. The labour ward was quite primitive, with small rooms and not much space. There were swing doors between each room, which meant midwives could move from one woman to another without going to the external corridor. Whilst this was useful for the midwives, the close proximity of the rooms and the gaps in the doors meant that couples could hear what was going on in the next room. This was not good for confidentiality and women would understandably get upset and frightened if they could hear another woman crying out.

The staff on the whole were great, and some of the midwives went out of their way to make me feel welcome. One or two were extra special and I immediately felt a bond with them and others I knew as they'd been out to work at Bramley as part of a staff rotation.

But I had to face a big culture shock in my new workplace. While at Bramley we'd concentrated on what the women wanted and worked with them at their pace, at Queens Park it was very different. This was largely because it was three times as busy and the midwives were really stretched to deliver all the care.

The approach from the midwives was very different too, as they often didn't have time to sit and be attentive as they were too busy dashing around caring for two women in labour at once.

Some midwives had been working in this environment all their career and I think had become conditioned into working in a certain way to help them to cope with the pressure. While most midwives were fantastic there would be the odd one who didn't appear to be putting the women in their care first.

I remember being alarmed to see a woman in advanced labour laid flat on her back on the bed, breathing ferociously on her gas and air. The door of the room was propped open and her midwife was stood at the door, chatting to the staff as they passed by. It seemed the woman needed her to be there and the midwife knew that, but also wanted to chat to her friends. Although this was a rare event it happened more than once and I couldn't help feeling sad. I didn't say anything to the midwife at all, which could be viewed as actually colluding with the practice, but I was the new girl and I needed to find a way of trying to influence the situation from within. I was fairly shy and non-confrontational, I didn't want to make any enemies, but at the same time I felt sorry for the women.

Whereas I'd previously cared for women who were deemed 'low risk' at Bramley Meade, many of the women at Queens Park had complex problems. Now I could be supporting women with diabetes and pre-eclampsia or women expecting twins or breech births. I knew the theory and during my training and early career I had some experience of caring for women with such conditions but I clearly needed to refresh my skills.

After working at Bramley where we were trying out all sorts of radical birthing plans I found some of the practices at Queens a little old-fashioned. Because of tradition, labouring women were treated as if they were ill, and 'procedures' ruled once more. I was surprised to see that women who'd just had a normal, uncomplicated birth would receive a bed bath by the staff before being wheeled to the postnatal ward on a trolley.

I had just left Bramley Meade where mothers had a bath after the birth, to freshen up, before moving to their bed independently if they felt comfortable enough to walk. I knew first-hand how comforting and soothing a warm bath could be after you've given birth. A bed bath paled in comparison. It seemed strange to wheel the women around like they were invalids and it was hard and unnecessary work for the staff.

Even more frustratingly I was asked again and again by new mums if they could just soak in the bath. After hours and hours of labour it was all they wanted.

'It's not allowed here, Sheena,' one midwife I'd occasionally worked with at Bramley warned. 'You'll get into trouble if you let them have one.'

It just seemed such a ridiculous rule. I really didn't want to make a fuss, in fact it took a great deal of courage to speak up, but believing I had the best interests of the women I was caring for at heart I kept mentioning it to the senior midwives. But to my frustration they told me repeatedly that Miss Davies wouldn't allow it just in case the woman had a fit in the bath.

'But these are healthy women,' I reasoned. 'I wouldn't put a woman in the bath if she was ill!'

It really pained me to go back and say no.

'Sorry, not right now,' I would say, before pausing for a moment. 'But ask me later once you're on the postnatal ward.'

I knew I shouldn't be disobeying my managers but I couldn't bear the thought of women struggling to feel clean.

So during the evening shifts and at weekends when there were less senior managers around I would help women to have their baths and then take them to the postnatal ward in a wheelchair. Unsurprisingly I did get caught by the fearful Miss Davies on two occasions.

'Byrom!' she'd yell, pointing her finger. 'My office. Now.'

Despite trying to explain my actions I got a real ticking off.

In hindsight I can see now that, principled or not, I was skating on thin ice. Eventually one of my dear colleagues took me aside.

'Sheena,' she said. 'I need to tell you something. Everyone is talking about you putting women in the bath.'

'But I'm not doing anything wrong!' I insisted.

'Actually, you are,' she said. 'And you could get struck off!'

Realising that I'd have to find other ways to convince staff, I decided to look for some evidence. In those days academic journals weren't as easily accessed and 'evidence-based care' wasn't a term we were used to. I really felt passionate about the issue so I decided to ring around other maternity units. Out of the six I called, all of them supported the use of bathing after birth if the woman felt well enough and there were no contraindications.

With this new knowledge I approached Mary, one of the senior midwives who I knew was influential.

'I actually agree with you,' she told me. 'Let me see what I can do.'

Mary must have spoken again with the managers as from then things started to change. Eventually it was agreed that women could have a bath as long as a member of staff was present in case a problem arose. It took about eighteen months but I got there in the end!

Maybe I was like a dog with a bone but the experiences I'd had at Bramley Meade had made me passionately believe that care should be centred around the individual needs of the woman. As midwives and doctors I felt we sometimes assumed a higher position than women – like we were the teachers and they were the pupils – but often women know what's best for their baby and themselves!

But there was no denying that being different or challenging practice didn't always do me favours – especially when Miss Davies was around. My intent was always to enhance care but even though I believed my practices were safe I was landing myself in trouble. I wasn't the only one, either – other colleagues who had been transferred after the closure also struggled with the procedures.

It was during this time that I learned about and joined the Association of Radical Midwives (ARM). This is a group of midwives who established themselves in the 1970s because they were unhappy with the medicalisation of childbirth and the unnecessary intervention in the childbirth process. Membership expanded and the group continues to influence practice successfully to this day. Although I didn't consider myself 'radical', I was keen to push boundaries and to stand up for what I believed to be right or what women said they needed. I found a sort of kinship within the membership of the group and I am still a member.

It wasn't just relatively minor issues like bathing policies that were different at Queens. I had been away from high-risk maternity care for a decade and during that time many changes had occurred that surprised and sometimes disturbed me – the rising use of epidurals for pain relief in labour being one.

Although epidurals were still not available to everyone due to reliance on adequate midwifery and anaesthetist staffing levels, it concerned me how increasingly frequently they were being administered.

Whilst there are various opinions and views on the risks and benefits of epidural, I can only speak from experience – experience of having one myself and experience of seeing how this intervention has radically changed the face of midwifery care and birth itself.

One of the disadvantages of an epidural is that it can slow down labour as it changes the shape of the pelvic floor. The physiology of labour is changed and the mother frequently needs drugs to speed her labour up. I also noticed that women seemed to find it harder to push with an epidural and as a result I saw more instrumental births, in which forceps or a ventouse are used to help the baby out.

Caring for a woman with an epidural for the first time reminded me of my nursing days when I had to move patients who were totally immobile. It would take two of us to move them with a 'lift and roll' action. This wasn't a problem, but it was so different to seeing women labour naturally, in control of their bodies.

I recall one woman who'd had an epidural with her first baby but really didn't want one the second time round. She had a traumatic first birth and when we discussed her records it seemed that the problems may have arisen from having the procedure. Beforehand she told me that she really didn't want to have an epidural this time, and made me promise not to relent.

Her labour progressed normally and when she got to the transition stage where her pain was most intensified she started to ask for one.

'I can't do it!' she begged. 'Please give me an epidural.'

'OK,' I said gently, 'But you told me earlier your really didn't want one.'

'Please, please, I can't do it!' she told me, her eyes filling with tears.

'Yes, you *can* do it,' I assured her. 'You are nearly there.'

I continued to support her and didn't leave her side. About three quarters of an hour later she gave birth to her daughter. I will never forget the joy on her face as she picked the baby up and pulled her up on to her chest. She was so happy.

'I did it!' she cried. 'I did it myself!'

As I went out of the room later I looked back to see the touching sight of mum and baby gazing at each other, all memories of the pain gone.

When women are well supported and are feeling the pains of labour, the body releases beta-endorphins, which are natural hormones that help to relieve pain and give a sense of euphoria. If the woman is afraid or feels anxious her body releases adrenaline, the 'fight-or-flight' hormone, which counteracts the endorphins, so that the pain intensifies.

Women who are affected by endorphins and experience the benefit can appear to be in an altered state of consciousness, or as some women describe it, 'on another planet'.

At Bramley Meade especially, I had the privilege of

witnessing this amazing process time and time again. Women feeling the pain, moving, moaning, crying out, rocking and shouting some more. Then, with unknown bursts of energy their baby is born and the immediate cessation of pain and rush of hormones is captured in their face with looks of pure joy. There is an everlasting sense of achievement, never to be forgotten – but I found that frequently epidural anaesthesia disturbs the whole process.

When I first went to Queens Park not everyone could have an epidural. There was only one obstetric anaesthetist and he could only administer one at a time. But within a few years there were more anaesthetists so if a woman really wanted one she could have it.

However, if I felt a woman was going to have her baby soon I'd try and support her through it. It's a fine line that all midwives have had to face and consider crossing. Women really do plead with midwives, especially during transition (the final, most difficult part of labour) when they are tired and the pain is at its worst.

Over the years I've heard women yell, 'Give me a section!' or 'Kill me now!' as they go through this part of labour. Some even try to get off the bed and leave. It's the hardest thing you ever do. The pain is unbelievable. It's on another level and sometimes women find it hard to deal with. But a skilled midwife can encourage women to get through that period because it is going to end.

Epidurals may have their place for *some* labours, but they can't replace the need for good supportive care and the constant attention of a birth companion.

Another new experience for me was being called out to

an event in the community as part of a 'flying squad' that despite its name meant travelling to an emergency situation by ambulance rather than helicopter. The flying squad was alerted if a woman was giving birth unexpectedly at home, was unable to make it to the hospital or had a problem arising at a home birth. These occasions were usually treated as emergencies but there were also less urgent events when the baby was already born (known as BBA – born before arrival) and the ambulance crew was already present and had reported mother and baby to be well.

Calls were received from the ambulance control or the community midwife and the shift coordinator on the labour ward would hastily arrange for a doctor and a midwife to go out with an ambulance to the appropriate address.

The ambulance would arrive at the hospital doors to pick up the staff who had to be ready and waiting with special bags and boxes containing the appropriate equipment and drugs, delivery packs and towels. The first time I attended a flying squad call-out it was in response to a message that a woman was in the advanced stages of labour and wanted to push.

It was a bitterly cold winter night and I was shivering as I waited nervously to be picked up at the hospital entrance, heavily laden as I was with bags and equipment. Within minutes the ambulance came swiftly to the door and I jumped in and off we went at a fair speed. The blue light was flashing but there was no siren, as at 3 a.m. the streets and roads were deathly quiet.

En route I asked questions of the crew, finding out more details about the situation awaiting us.

'All we know is that a call came in from the woman herself, saying she can't move,' they told me. My stomach churned with a sense of anticipation as I wondered what we would find.

Eventually we turned into a dark street on a large estate where some of the houses were boarded up. With the dim street lighting I felt like we were in a war zone. Finding the house, we let ourselves in. My first impression was that the house was every bit as cold inside as it was outside. Clearly the walls were very thin and there was no insulation.

Following the sounds of crying I rushed upstairs, where through an open door I saw a toddler stood up in a cot, crying but unattended. He looked cold.

The next room was a small box room where the child's mother Kara was laid on her back, obviously in labour and whimpering. She looked at us with a pale, pinched face and said nothing. The room was barren, small and empty, except the bed, which had just one thin blanket as a cover.

'Kara, my name is Sheena, I'm the midwife,' I told her, bending down and giving her a reassuring hug. 'Don't worry, we're here now and we'll look after you. Now I'm just going to listen to your baby's heart . . .'

As I spoke I could see my own breath in the air. It was freezing. One of the ambulance crew was busy trying to console the crying child in the next room and the other stayed close by me, helping.

Within minutes Kara was ready to push and in the dimmed light I could see the baby's head emerging easily.

'Aarggh! Help me, PLEASE!' Kara cried and I stroked her face to try and comfort her. Just minutes later she gave birth to a beautiful baby girl who arrived into the cold room literally steaming. Quickly I wrapped her up in a towel and snuggled her up inside my fleece to keep her warm until the placenta had been removed. Normally I would have immediately passed the baby to the mum, as the warmest place for the baby to be is usually close to its mother's body. But it was so cold, and Kara was shaking and shivering too. Searching the house the ambulance men managed to gather some coats to put on the bed to help keep her and the baby warm.

Kara seemed very sad and didn't speak very much. It concerned me greatly that the house was freezing and she was there on her own. I sat with her for some time helping her to feed her baby. She had a few clothes ready and we dressed the baby together.

'Is there anyone who might come and look after you and your children for a while?' I asked. She turned her head away.

'It would be better if you had someone close by,' I said gently. Reluctantly she gave me the number of a relative who I called and asked to come round. I wanted to help her more but wasn't sure how.

I didn't ask her about her personal circumstances but I wondered, if she still had a partner, if he were away in the army or navy? Yet usually there would be someone else there to help – a friend, mum, an aunty or a sister. It was her isolation that saddened me. Kara's sister-in-law arrived just before we left and agreed to care for her for a couple of days. Kara didn't want or need to go to hospital so when we had checked mum and baby were fine and warm, we left.

It wouldn't be the first or last time I'd see a situation that was less than ideal, and it was never something I got used to. I often thought about the things I had seen during my working day when I got home, and in bed at night, and some incidences have never left me. It's the desperation that affected me most, the sheer inability for some women and families to emerge even slightly from the plight they are in, from the drudgery and darkness of their everyday lives. As a young girl I had witnessed my mum helping others less fortunate by doing something small for them that made a massive difference, like sharing her food. But my gift was to be as kind as I could, and to try to influence women's self-esteem in a non-patronising way.

As I got to grips with my work at Queens Park, life at home was as busy as ever. With four young ones and a family home to run it was never going to be easy. But thankfully my friends Jill, Pat and Katie were always on hand to help out with babysitting and school pick-ups. We couldn't have managed without them.

Our children were growing fast and seemingly had more hobbies than we did! There was always something going on. Anna and James loved music and drama and were members of amateur dramatic societies. There was piano, singing lessons, ballet, athletics and sport. Anna excelled at dance and was chosen to take part in competitions (dance festivals), which was like entering into another world. James was proving to be gifted at piano and in fact now earns a living as a pianist. Tom preferred football, rugby and wrestling!

Olivia meanwhile was both a girl's girl *and* a tomboy, singing along cutely to *Les Mis* and running around the garden after a football.

The house and garden would often be besieged by the children's friends, the neighbours and cousins, with both my sisters' and Paul's brothers' kids coming round for play-days and family get-togethers. All in all there was never a dull moment.

Mum was still living with Anne, and it was becoming more apparent as the months went by that the stroke had permanently damaged her speech. Poor Mum. Her vibrant life was cut short through this cruel and frustrating condition. It was so hard for her, but my sisters and Aunty Pat and Marion tried hard to make her life more tolerable.

Mum was as brave as ever, trying hard to be positive when she was now cruelly a prisoner in her own body. Her eyes were so expressive and knowing her so well we could often tell how she was feeling. She did sometimes cry loudly, and we would hold her close.

She would try to tell us things, often repeating: 'Do you know why?' That was all she could say. Over time we learned to interpret what she was trying to tell us, but much of it was guesswork. The days must have been so long for Mum, and I often wonder what she thought, as she could never tell us.

After some time working on day duty at Queens Park the option came up for me to work some night shifts.

I liked being on nights once more as not only did it fit in with my family, but also the wards were often peaceful and

I had more opportunities to spend time caring for the labouring women.

One night I was looking after a woman who was in very early labour. She was on her own as her husband had gone off to see to their other child, so I sat with her, supporting her and rubbing her back when her contractions came.

She was drifting in and out of sleep and using gas and air from time to time. Well, I don't know quite what happened but the next moment I was aware of my name being called. Jerking awake, I opened my eyes. It was my colleague Diane who had appeared at the door looking for me.

'Sheena!' she hissed. 'You're asleep!'

She was interrupted by the woman, who, rather touchingly, appeared to have had her arm around me! 'Sssh,' she chastised. 'She's tired!' It seemed her maternal instincts were kicking in already. I was absolutely horrified and, after apologising profusely, I carried on caring for her with a newfound alertness. I was so embarrassed even though she reassured me that my eyes were closed for literally a few seconds.

My colleagues never let it drop and for many years to come they teased me mercilessly. While it makes a funny story, it wasn't my finest moment. In my later years as a manager there were occasions when I had to deal with staff who had been sleeping on duty and, although in those incidents their falling to sleep was intentional, I am only too aware of how bad it was to nod off, even if only momentarily.

Chapter 10

The elderly gentleman shuffled awkwardly from foot to foot.

'It's about one of your mothers,' he said, glancing nervously over his shoulder to make sure the coast was clear. 'She's outside the hospital selling drugs.'

My colleague and I glanced at each other with shocked but knowing looks. What were the chances that he was talking about Adele – a mum in her early twenties who had been missing for the last hour after 'popping out' for a cigarette.

For the last thirty minutes we'd been scouring the hospital for her to no avail. She was neither in the smokers' room nor the courtyard in the middle of the hospital, and with staff having to bottlefeed her day-old baby in her absence we were worried.

The description certainly fitted and after thanking the man, a patient on another ward, we kept our eyes peeled for Adele's return.

Ten minutes later she sloped back on to the ward looking completely unfazed. We had no choice but to say something.

'We're not going to report you,' I said. 'But you can't be selling drugs in the hospital.'

'It wasn't in the hospital. It was outside,' she replied bolshily, but eventually agreed not to do it again before being discharged the following day.

There were certainly some interesting moments on the postnatal ward – where, eighteen months into my stint at Queens Park, I was now working. The change in department came as part of a rotation plan for midwives to ensure that our skills were maintained in all areas of midwifery.

'Welcome to Caesar's Palace,' announced my new manager, Sister Wardle.

This was her tongue-in-cheek reference to the fact she believed too many Caesarean sections were being performed at the hospital, causing her an increasing amount of work. She was probably right although the number of operative births has almost doubled since her day!

Just like the labour ward, postnatal was very busy as there were many medical interventions. As well as post-op care for women who'd had Caesarean sections and epidurals, there were always small babies to be fed at specific times. Likewise there were often babies who weren't feeding well or whose mothers had raised temperatures during labour, and who needed regular antibiotics as a preventative measure to ward off potential infections.

It was demanding but rewarding work and while there was always plenty to do, there was also an air of cheeriness as the women enjoyed their first days of motherhood.

While most women were straightforward and polite

they inevitably had their little moments from time to time. A common problem was women getting fed up with waiting to take their babies home.

Although midwives today can check mums and babies over and then send them home, in the early nineties it was down to the paediatrician to discharge the baby. Relying on doctors could be problematic as sick babies were prioritised, meaning the others often had to wait.

With mothers keeping their babies in cots beside their beds the postnatal ward was often very noisy. On day two or three of their stay women wanted to go home with their babies. They often complained of lack of sleep due to other babies in the room crying.

'I'm just not waiting any more,' they'd announce on the verge of tears and we'd have to reassure them.

While I was working on the postnatal ward, Pauline Quinn was busy trying to establish new models of care to provide at least a small amount of continuity to women. It was her belief that women shouldn't have to see so many midwives during their childbirth experience and they should have their care covered by just a few.

I was still working part-time at this stage but was very interested in Pauline's idea and how it would work within our unit. Keen to find out more I read a book by a highly regarded midwife called Caroline Flint, who encouraged a nurturing approach to midwifery and highlighted inadequacies in the maternity care system in England at the time.

Caroline had introduced a scheme called 'Know Your Midwife' and I attended a seminar she ran on the topic where she explained the idea behind the innovation. Like

Mrs Quinn, Caroline wanted to try to reduce the number of different midwives a woman came into contact with during pregnancy, as she thought it led to confusion for the woman and reduced satisfaction. She said that if we organised ourselves differently, it could work.

The seminar inspired me to learn more so I spoke to Sister Wardle and asked her if I could try to help implement the concept on our ward. Sister Wardle was skeptical.

'You're wasting your time, it'll never work,' she said. 'But go ahead if you want to.'

Undeterred, I tried to think how I could make a difference on the postnatal ward. I could certainly start by ensuring women at least knew the names of the staff, so my friend Angela and I devised a huge board and took photographs of all the midwives and nurses who worked on the ward. It went down well and although it didn't actually change the number of staff women saw, it was a small step for women to know who their midwife was!

I was busy working on other ideas to implement when a new opportunity came up – a community midwife role in the Ribble Valley where I lived.

It was one afternoon in 1993 as I was leaving the hospital after a busy early shift when I bumped into one of my colleagues, Claire, who worked on another ward.

'Are you applying for the community midwife post they've been advertising?' she asked.

'I don't know anything about it,' I admitted.

Community midwives were quite separate from the hospital midwives and provided maternity services in GP surgeries and in women's homes. They were all midwifery sisters, although the word 'sister' was now being phased out due to its association with nursing.

Claire got me thinking. There were two posts advertised: one in Blackburn and the other in the Ribble Valley.

At this point Olivia was a little girl, four in fact, and to work full-time would be hard. Then there were Anna and James who were teenagers and driving me mad. Their school was very strict and I was frequently called in to see the headmaster when they were playing up (James's crimes included having leather shoelaces in his sports trainers as opposed to normal fabric ones). On top of that I'd often have to get in the middle of them as they fought like cat and dog.

But the job spec revealed the post holder would be working nine till five with the odd weekend and nights on call. Although my workload would double it would mean less unsociable hours and more evenings with my family. It would also be a promotion and much more responsibility. I went home and had a long chat with Paul.

'Sounds like a good opportunity,' he said. 'I can help with Olivia and at least she's at school now.' He also pointed out that the chance might not arise again any time soon.

The more I thought about it the more enthused I felt. It would be wonderful to work in the community and to see and support families at home. Most of all I was excited at the prospect of home births! I could go back to 'catching' babies in a non-medical environment like Bramley Meade. By the end of the evening I really wanted to go for the job.

I applied the following day and was invited for an interview, which was gruelling to say the least.

There was a panel of three: Miss Davies, the manager from the labour ward, Mrs Quinn and the community midwife manager, Miss Harris, a tall, dark, heavy-set woman aged about forty-five. I'd never had an interview at that level before and when I walked into the room my knees were audibly knocking.

'Tell me about yourself,' Mrs Quinn began.

Once more, true to form, I opened my mouth but I just couldn't speak! My mouth was all dried up with the nerves and after a long pause they brought me some water.

After a big swig I attempted to speak again. I told them all about my career so far, my expanding experience as a midwife and the project I had begun to instigate on the postnatal ward. I was enthused by the nods of one of the panel members but less encouraged by the scowls of the other two!

I left feeling very unsure about how well I'd done. But later that day I was absolutely over the moon to learn that I had been successful. A friend of mine, Caroline, had also got the Blackburn post so there were celebrations all round.

It was to prove a significant time in my career and a massive learning curve.

Working as a community midwife I was allocated various GP clinics in the Ribble Valley, mainly, to my delight, in Clitheroe, the lovely market town where I used to live. I was now working with a petite midwife called Janet Jackson, who was very experienced and taught me the ropes with care and enthusiasm. She was to become a great friend to me. She introduced me to the GPs, their receptionists (sometimes surprisingly scary) and to other members of the surgery teams.

Janet and I each shared half the midwifery care for the GPs in Clitheroe and each week we would see the same women at their antenatal appointments. Then if one of us was on holiday, we would cover for each other. My working day was nine till five but the hours were flexible and I often worked more on one day and less on another.

The work consisted of running antenatal clinics on the surgery premises, which women would attend for their check-up in pregnancy. Although sometimes, during the early days, the GPs would be in attendance, very often I'd see up to twenty women in one session on my own. It was a very busy time but I thoroughly enjoyed these clinics, building up good relationships with women as I saw them week after week.

After the clinics I had a list of home visits, obtained from the hospital the night before. The visits were to women who had had their baby and needed a check, or to those who were pregnant and having problems, such as raised blood pressure.

Working in the community meant I had to learn a whole new approach. I was practising more on my own now so there was a lot more responsibility. If I missed anything no one else would be checking later on, so I needed to be extra vigilant. I was also a guest in the homes of the families I was visiting, and had to remember that.

The Ribble Valley was a rural community with vast areas of countryside and sometimes there was a great deal of driving involved as I'd travel ten to twenty miles from one postnatal check to another. On most days I'd drive through the most fabulous scenery, rippling green hills and groups of ancient, majestic trees. On bright spring mornings or glorious summer days this was heavenly – however, the journey was considerably less pleasant when the heavens opened, a gale blew or snow fell. Knowing that one thing I could not rely on was the great British weather, I never set off without a waterproof mac and a pair of wellies in the boot of my car, no matter how sunny it appeared.

One particularly grim and stormy day I travelled eighteen miles in the pouring rain to a remote farm in Slaidburn, a small village in the Forest of Bowland. As was the case with many of the farms I visited, the bumpy, uneven road to the farmhouse wound through open farmland. Eventually I met a five-bar gate, which was closed to prevent the animals getting out.

The rain was hammering against my windscreen and, as I clambered out, the wind caught my car door violently. It took every effort to get to the gate to open it, return to my car, drive through, then go back out into the pelting rain to close it once more.

Scrabbling back into my Honda Civic I breathed a sigh of relief – that is until, to my utter dismay, I came to gate number two and had to get out and fight the elements once more. Two further gates later and I pulled up outside the farmhouse, soaked to the bone and filthy.

Thankfully the farmer wasn't at all put out to open the door to a drowned rat purporting to be his spouse's midwife.

'Come on in and get dried!' he boomed. Stepping in the door I immediately felt warm and welcomed.

I loved visiting farmhouses as they always felt cosy and there were almost always delicious smells of home baking filling the kitchen. The sense of family tradition and basic living was comforting.

Glenda, the farmer's wife, had just had her third baby so we sat by the fire chatting while I attempted to get dry. As was usual I checked her and the baby and then tried to help a little, offering to hang out the washing or do the odd job. This was typical of the kind of relationship I had with the women I visited in the community. Having seen them all the way through their pregnancy it was almost like you'd become a friend to them. They welcomed me like one of the family, I got to know them well and they'd often confide in me if something was bothering them. On this occasion Glenda seemed fine – relaxed and happy and enjoying time with her baby.

From my experience this laid-back attitude was fairly typical of farmers' wives. Whether I went to attend their home births or saw them before or after the birth, they really seemed to take it all in their stride. Perhaps it was because they saw animals giving birth every day and just viewed it as a normal part of nature?

This most definitely seemed to be the case with Jill, a farmer's wife pregnant with her third baby who wanted a home birth. I hadn't been the midwife for her first two but I'd seen her all the way through her pregnancy this time and knew her really well. She lived on a busy farm and in the lead up to her baby's arrival I could tell she was looking forward to giving birth, as being pregnant was clearly getting in the way of her work!

When she called to say she might be in labour it wasn't a total surprise when she asked me not to come for a while.

'I'm having contractions but I want to see to the cows and get my other jobs done,' she told me candidly. 'Come in a few hours.'

'OK,' I replied. 'But I'd really like to come now and check your baby. I'll just hang around and won't get in the way.'

When I arrived at the farmhouse it was clear Jill was in labour but that wasn't about to stop her from doing her daily chores. Once I'd checked her and her baby, off she continued in a cleaning frenzy. One minute she was cleaning buckets out in the yard, the next she was hanging out her washing or helping with the animals. I offered to assist her but she wouldn't let me lift a finger.

It was actually great to see her so active. She'd stop occasionally for me to carry out some more checks and I could tell her labour was getting more advanced by her breathing. Eventually I spied her through the window, leaning over her brush, puffing and blowing.

'Do you need me?' I asked.

'No, I'm fine!' she insisted.

As her contractions got closer and closer I guided her upstairs as she wanted to give birth in the marital bed.

'I think I'm ready to push now,' she said, so I quickly called another midwife to assist. Her husband was around but didn't come in, as he wanted to carry on with his farm duties.

Meanwhile Jill had a wonderful labour. She only got on the bed at the last minute to push out her beautiful baby girl. She looked so proud when we tucked her up with her baby and her husband brought in their two little boys. 'Mummy, when did she come?' they asked, wide-eyed, as they scrambled up on the bed.

The whole thing just felt like it was part of everyday life and as I left hours later to continue with my work for the day I felt a warm glow glancing at the happy family snuggled together. No fuss, no anxieties, no trips to hospital.

It was no surprise when I returned the next day to find Jill back on her feet, busy breastfeeding her baby, keeping everything shipshape. The house had quickly returned to its usual hub of activity with the baby just fitting in.

Another of my responsibilities as a community midwife was to provide antenatal education or 'parentcraft' sessions, where women or couples came to learn about what to expect and were taught skills such as how to feed their babies.

I found this quite nerve-wracking at first, as while I had a wealth of knowledge on the topics we were discussing I certainly wasn't used to imparting it to a room full of people! It was daunting, particularly as the sessions were well attended and I was quite shy.

It was a confidence issue really and I had to get used to it. At my first session Janet was with me, having coached me to get to that point. Although it went OK I felt I was a bit ropey.

To help improve my confidence I attended some sessions taught by Clare Harding, who held private National Childbirth Trust (NCT) eight-week courses for expectant parents in Blackburn. Clare was well respected, popular and a fabulous NCT teacher. Couples would go to her home and she'd sit in the middle and feed them homemade cake whilst talking about having babies, in a very different way than I was used to!

As the weeks passed I saw the couples build up wonderful relationships with each other, and with Clare. I learned so much from her and she taught me that while we as health professionals think we are there to deliver all the knowledge, it is actually a two-way process. Women knew their bodies well and had valuable information to share with us, too. Clare influenced the way I held my lessons from then on, and the content of her sessions taught me much more about childbirth from a different perspective.

As well as my new responsibilities hosting antenatal sessions, my new role also meant that – as I'd hoped – I was frequently attending home births.

One of the most memorable home births I attended was working alongside one of my friends, Yvonne, who was an independent midwife.

Being an independent midwife meant that Yvonne was self-employed, instead of working for the NHS. Sometimes women are unhappy with the models of maternity care in the NHS or they want a more personalised service and midwives too sometimes choose to work in a way where they are more autonomous and not restrained by the rules and policies that exist within public sector organisations. Yvonne and I had similar philosophies of midwifery and used to sometimes share our frustrations with current maternity services.

On this occasion Yvonne had been employed by a lady called Amanda Parker, whose family lived in a majestic ancestral home called Browsholme Hall in the Forest of Bowland. The Hall dates back to 1507 and has been in the possession of the same family ever since.

Yvonne had cared for Amanda when she had her first baby, who was a breech presentation and who was born in hospital by Caesarean section. When she fell pregnant for the second time Amanda wanted Yvonne to be her midwife again. This time she was planning to have the baby at home – a historical moment for the family as there hadn't been a baby born at the house for a hundred years!

There were some important considerations to be made here, as when a woman has had a previous Caesarean she would normally be advised to have her second baby in hospital where medical assistance is available should complications arise. However, the decision ultimately belongs to the women in question and Yvonne was supporting Amanda in her choice. To cover all eventualities, Yvonne was liaising with the supervisor of midwives and consultant obstetrician at our maternity unit. Her GP would be present and a plan was in place should she need to be transferred into hospital. Yvonne also asked for support from an NHS midwife during Amanda's labour. When the community midwife manager discussed this at one of our meetings I was asked to help out.

When Amanda went into labour in the early afternoon Yvonne called me and told me to head over. Grabbing my kit I jumped in my car and set off to the address I'd been given.

Making my way up the driveway I was absolutely astounded by the size of the place. It was 6 p.m. and as dusk fell on the hall I was immediately struck by how regal and grand it was. I wondered how many other midwives had arrived at this building over the centuries, as it was clearly steeped in history. After I'd parked up I walked up to the front door where I rang the huge bell.

A smartly dressed gentleman greeted me at the door (I assumed he was the butler – I wasn't about to ask) and he walked me through a massive entrance hall.

We passed a suit of armour and a huge fireplace and everywhere I looked there were enormous old paintings on the walls. Following him upstairs we walked past several stained-glass windows. I was just mesmerised as I took in the lavish, exquisite surroundings.

Eventually we came to a stunning room with ancient, dark wood furniture and lavish fittings that looked like the perfect setting for a period drama – apart from the 500 square feet of polythene that Amanda's husband had spread across the floor.

'I don't know what he thought was going to happen!' Amanda commented later.

Yvonne was busy attending to Amanda. The centrepiece of the room was a grand four-poster bed, on which Amanda was moving around and working through her labour.

Her labour continued for a further hour after I arrived, with Amanda giving birth to her son Roland just after 7 p.m. with no problems or complications. I stayed for a while until mother and baby were settled, then headed home to prepare for work.

I was to visit Amanda and Roland at Browsholme a few times after the birth and it was always the highlight of my day. I was always itching to look around the house but sadly our meetings always took place in her kitchen.

The house is now open to the public and I cycle past it most weekends. I'd really like to wander around and soak up the atmosphere, imagining family life there, not to mention reminiscing with Amanda about the night her son was born.

Yvonne isn't practising as a midwife now but we meet up from time to time and often chat about her days as an independent midwife. As she says herself, she has never forgotten the huge adrenaline rush, excitement and anticipation of being called to a home birth and the memories still bring a lump to her throat.

As well as home births there was another development in midwifery that I was starting to witness in my new role. During the 1990s a new, exciting kind of birth was coming into fashion as women began to give birth in water. I'd read about water births in journals and had seen study days on the topic advertised. I knew that having a warm, deep bath helped women with their contractions but that was as far as my practical experience went and I was yet to see a baby born underwater.

Then one day I received a call from Janet to say that one of her mothers-to-be, a lady called Helen, not only wanted a water birth but had her heart set on having it at home.

We were both excited by this prospect, so after reporting in with our managers we went to Helen's house together to discuss her request further.

Helen had previously had her two-year-old daughter

Anna at home and knew exactly how she wanted things this time around.

'I don't want my GP there,' she told us. 'I want it to be cosy, just me, the midwife, my husband and my little girl Anna.'

When it came to discussing the possibility of a water birth, she was equally determined.

'I've researched it all,' she said firmly. 'I know how it will happen, I know what pool I want and I just want to run the logistics past you.'

'OK,' Janet replied. 'We'll go back and discuss it with our manager and get back to you.'

Back at Queens Park we were given the green light for Helen's water birth and our manager, Miss Harris, who was keen for us to be well prepared, sent us to get some training. A few weeks later, Janet and I attended a study day with Janet Balaskas, the founder of the Active Birth Movement and a big advocate of water births.

It was a very informative day and gave us a real insight into how to care for a woman in water. There were lots of important factors such as maintaining the temperature of the water and how to check everything was OK while the woman was immersed. We also met some midwives from other units who were already facilitating water births and they shared knowledge with us too. The highlight of the day was Janet showing us slides of photos of women giving birth under water. We were amazed.

Finally we went to Blackpool maternity unit where pools were used regularly for labour and birth and where the midwives were proficient in supporting women who chose to use water.

The midwives there gave us copies of the guidelines they followed to help ensure mother and baby were as safe as possible. We had long chats about the logistics of using water and we found that the whole team there was encouraging and positive.

'It's an amazing experience,' one midwife told me. 'The water makes such a difference.'

Janet and I went away feeling very excited about Helen's impending water birth.

With all this new information Janet and I set about writing our own local guidelines about what we'd do for Helen's forthcoming birth. It was quite an event for our maternity unit and we had regular meetings to discuss it. The supervisors of midwives and the management team were all aware of what was going on. We also passed on all the information to the other community midwives so they could support us if necessary.

As it happened Janet was going to be away on holiday around Helen's due date, so I agreed to provide all the on-call cover as 'first' midwife, and some of my colleagues agreed to be backup.

At last, Helen's much-anticipated labour began and, following instructions, I immediately called the maternity unit and informed the supervisor on call.

It was a weekend day, and after saying goodbye to my family, I jumped in my car and travelled to Helen's with a big smile on my face. I was all set for another fascinating twist in my career but I also felt slightly apprehensive. I'd never delivered a baby under water before!

Helen, her husband John and their little girl were waiting

for me and busily preparing the pool. Water was being pumped from the kitchen tap, and the pool had been set up in the dining room. John had already had several practice runs to ensure there were no hiccoughs on the special day.

When I checked Helen she was definitely in labour and ready to immerse herself in the water. I called Sue, the midwife who was on call as backup that day, and also checked in with Mrs Quinn, who was supervisor on call that day.

'Everything is on track,' I reassured her. I also informed the delivery suite staff at the hospital.

'Good news, Sheena. Now make sure you call if you need anything,' they said. 'And let us know as soon as the baby is born.' It was comforting to know my colleagues were supporting me even just at the end of a telephone.

Carefully John and I helped Helen into the pool. She visibly sighed as the water worked its magic on her contractions and soon we were joined by her daughter Anna who hung on to the side of the pool, chatting away to her mummy. Anna was also keen to 'help' us when we checked the water temperature and even got in herself for a short while.

As Helen's contractions got stronger and more intense, Anna was ushered off to bed by her father.

It was amazing watching Helen in the water. Her eyes remained closed most of the time and she moved and swayed in her own little world.

When each contraction came she moaned and moved until it passed. I sat nearby and watched in wonderment. I never failed to be in awe of women as they progressed magnificently through one contraction after another – especially after I'd done it myself and knew how hard it was!

Sue and I watched and listened, staying quiet so as not to disturb the atmosphere of the incredibly intimate space we were in.

The only interruption we made was when I had to listen to the baby's heartbeat. Unfortunately I didn't have a water-proof sonicaid (the doppler gadget that picks up the heart-beat) so this meant Helen had to stand up. But each time she took it in her stride then settled back into her labour.

The room was very tranquil as Helen's deep, controlled breaths intertwined with the ticking of the clock and the faint music playing in the background.

We drank tea and waited for her cue.

'I think I want to push,' she eventually said.

Sue and I moved closer while Helen knelt in the pool and seemed to be positioning herself. Under the water we could see the baby's head emerging, and we held our breath.

'This is it!' I thought. With a strong push, Helen forced her baby's body out easily. She gathered him gently and swiftly and brought his face up to the surface, holding him delicately on the surface of the water and watching his face as he blinked and looked at her.

'Hello, little man,' she whispered. It was a beautiful moment. We checked baby's breathing and all was well, and then left mother and son to become acquainted. Helen didn't need any stitches so we had a cup of tea to celebrate.

Then with all the post-birth checks completed and normal I called my colleagues at the hospital and Mrs Quinn to let them know.

Finally, after lots of hugs and words of congratulations, Sue and I left them to get to know the baby boy they'd named Scott. We had to head back to the hospital to complete some records and drop the placenta off but first we sat together in the car for a while.

'Wow,' I said. 'How amazing, how utterly amazing!' We felt proud of ourselves, too.

Chapter 11

The following day, still giddy with excitement after witnessing my first-ever water birth, I called in to see how Helen and baby Scott were doing.

Helen was still very excited by her achievement and had even called the local press to report on Scott's birth – the first birth using a water pool in the area!

She asked if I'd be in the photo as well, so after checking that was OK with my seniors, I duly posed with them, smiling for a photo that was published in the local paper.

I didn't think much more about my five minutes of fame until a couple of weeks later when my direct line manager Miss Harris returned from her holiday and bleeped me on my two-way walkie-talkie.

'Number twenty-one, I need to see you urgently, over and out,' came the message. The tone of her voice concerned me.

'Is there something wrong? Over and out,' I asked.

'Just come in to my office quickly,' she replied. At the time I was miles away from the hospital and busy in a clinic. I didn't know what to think and for the rest of the afternoon

I felt sick. Had I done something wrong? What could it be that was so urgent?

As soon as I had finished my work for the day, I headed to Blackburn as fast as I could to meet the boss. Miss Harris made me feel uneasy at the best of times and I knew she wasn't my biggest fan.

When I walked into her office she was sat behind her desk with her back to the window. I saw that in front of her on her desk she had the newspaper cutting about Helen's water birth.

'Have you had a nice holiday?' I asked. She ignored the question.

'OK, I've called you in because of this,' she said, wafting the newspaper at me. 'Explain yourself. What is this all about?'

When I opened my mouth to answer she interrupted.

'Before you start, I'm very worried about the way you cared for this woman,' she continued, opening up a folder with my delivery notes in. 'You didn't give the syntometrine as and when we agreed. Why?'

Syntometrine is a drug used to help the placenta to be delivered, which Helen had wanted to have. But when we had been drafting our guidelines there had been a debate about when it was to be given, before or after Helen got out of the pool. Usually the injection was given just as the baby's body is about to be born, but as this wouldn't be possible with a water birth it had been suggested that it was given after the birth, just as Helen was about to leave the pool, giving it time to work.

But at the time Helen had wanted to wait until she got

out the water, so that's what we did. It was of no significance really and I was horrified that this was even mentioned.

'Helen wanted it that way,' I began, attempting to defend myself.

'Do you always do everything people want?' she replied. 'This newspaper, what a spectacle! Putting yourself in the public eye.'

'But I asked permission from Mrs Quinn, the supervisor on call!' I explained in disbelief.

'Oh?' said Miss Harris. 'I didn't know that.'

She was starting to backtrack but it was too late. Her accusing tone had really winded me and before I could stop myself I started to cry.

I'd felt so upbeat and proud of myself after Helen's water birth and these recriminations now were such a blow. It was the last reaction I expected. There was no mention of the fact that all had gone well, mother and baby were healthy and Helen was totally happy about her birth. Let alone that the story in the press was positive for the maternity service. I didn't have a hanky on me and as I tried to wipe my tears away with my fingers she remained silent. She didn't get up from her seat, offer me a tissue or say sorry for upsetting me. I was so embarrassed that I stood up and turned to leave.

'Where are you going?' she demanded.

'I'm leaving,' I replied, my hand shaking as I closed the door behind me. I never heard anything more about the incident, and she never tried to talk to me about it again.

In another blow I found out later that a particular midwife who knew how to keep in Miss Harris's good books had kindly saved the paper and brought it for her to see. She didn't know that I'd checked everything out with my seniors prior to being photographed, which was one of the rules, and I suspected she was trying to drop me in it.

In my career I remember the wonderful midwives but I also recall others who could be deliberately intimidating and controlling, creating a culture of fear. It still puzzles me. When I was eventually promoted to team leader and then to a manager I used my own experiences of good and bad from previous leaders to help to shape my own style. I tried hard to lead with encouragement and with positive actions, as I don't believe people flourish with intimidation and criticism.

At home there were further testing times as the children grew older and rebelled further. When they weren't bickering Anna and James were thick as thieves and instead of doing their homework they would devise cunning plans to skive off. In one ingenious ruse James would start playing the piano, creating a diversion, while Anna sneaked out the door. Then James would head into the kitchen under the pretence of making a sandwich and bolt out the back door to join her. To this day they are proud as punch of this trick and we always laugh when they recount it.

However, when they were in the midst of their terrible teens it was truly trying. If I came home after a hard day's work, arguments within the family – whether they were due to Paul being a grump or the kids being plain naughty – drove me mad.

Not one to stay and argue I'd just walk out the door to cool down. It usually did the trick.

While like every family we had our ups and downs, we also were incredibly close and the rows never festered for long and were soon forgotten. I found sounding off to my friends who had older children really helped.

'It's perfectly normal,' Katie, my old friend from the labour ward assured me. 'I went through all this with my son so you mustn't worry.'

It was reassuring to hear, even if it didn't help when I was in the midst of it.

Most Friday afternoons Miss Harris held a meeting with all the available community midwives, at the hospital in Blackburn. It was at one of those meetings that she read out a letter from a lady called Emma.

Emma was thirty-six weeks' pregnant (in other words, four weeks before her due date) and was managing a hostel for the homeless in Swansea. Her letter detailed how she was about to move to Clitheroe and wanted a home birth, as she'd originally planned to have in Swansea.

But at that particular time local guidance for midwives stipulated that women wanting a home birth would need to have had a normal birth previously. This was Emma's first child so in theory she would have to have her baby in hospital.

Miss Harris instructed Janet or I to go and see Emma to discuss her plans, so the following day I went to see her at home.

I liked Emma immediately. I thought she had a wonderful

approach to childbirth and I listened intently as she explained that having her baby at home fitted in with her philosophy of life.

She informed me that in Swansea the midwives and GP had been supportive of her planned home birth and how she'd been shocked to learn that in Clitheroe the policy was different. But it was Emma's choice at the end of the day.

'I'll speak to my manager and supervisor and if it's all agreed I will be on call for you and will try to be there for your baby's birth,' I told her. Back at the hospital I chatted to Miss Harris about Emma's plan and we agreed that it was important to provide good support to Emma.

After that I saw Emma every week. Even though we only had four or five meetings we got on really well and I grew very fond of her.

It was an April morning when Emma rang in the early hours to say she'd started with her contractions. They were coming regularly and building up in strength so I quickly got dressed and headed out.

On the drive over I saw it was a beautiful morning and as the sun came up I felt excited for Emma and her husband Sonam.

When I arrived at the house Emma was already in her space, meditating quietly. Sonam was there and also her best friend, Anne. Sonam didn't speak much English and was keeping himself busy around the house.

As the hours passed, Emma was obviously progressing in labour. She was clearly working hard with her contractions, closing her eyes when the waves came, but in between her face was relaxed and happy. Anne was rubbing her back and holding her and the room and whole house was very peaceful and serene.

Emma was doing well and her progress in labour continued to be perfect as she showed signs of coming to the final stages. The second midwife, Linda, had arrived and was sat quietly nearby as I did a further vaginal examination.

At this point Emma was standing as I moved around her, keen not to disturb her too much. I noted that her cervix was nine centimetres dilated but then during the examination her waters broke. Linda then used a sonicaid transmitter to pick up the pulses of the baby's heartbeat. Immediately we glanced at each other. To our alarm the baby's heartbeat was only sixty beats per minute (the normal range is between 110 to 150 bpm). This sometimes happens briefly after membranes rupture but as we continued to listen there was no recovery and the heartbeat remained worryingly slow. The baby was in distress, and needed to be born.

Linda immediately sprang into action, alerting the relevant emergency services. The flying squad was on its way, bringing an obstetrician, a paediatrician and another midwife. Linda also called the local GP who arrived within minutes. Emma was clearly alarmed and I concentrated on supporting her, knowing full well the gravity of the situation.

'What's happening?' she asked, her eyes boring into mine.

I explained as best I could, adding that there was no apparent reason why her baby's heartbeat was so low.

Before long the emergency team arrived and after a full assessment the decision was made to transfer Emma into hospital. However, with the risk the baby could be born en route (and therefore need resuscitation) we needed to wait for a second ambulance. With the hospital approximately twelve miles away, this caused another anxious wait.

Sonam was clearly confused and worried and with him not speaking English I wasn't sure whether he was fully aware of the seriousness of the situation.

I was holding Emma as she worked hard in my arms, by now trying to push her baby out. The paediatrician waited expectantly in an adjacent bedroom with his equipment set out. The baby's heartbeat continued to beat slowly and glancing up I saw the obstetrician's face showed signs of anguish. She, like me, just wanted the baby to be born. My instincts were telling me to put Emma in my car and quickly drive her to the hospital but I wasn't allowed to do that. The clocked ticked on as we waited until eventually the second ambulance arrived and we set off in convoy to Queens Park.

As we raced through the towns on the way to the hospital I sat in the first ambulance with Emma and the obstetrician. Emma was propped up on the stretcher and Sonam was in front of her, clearly anxious and unsure of what was going on. As I continued to monitor Emma and her baby with some difficulty, I could feel her eyes glued to my face, looking for any sign that would reveal her baby's fate.

Inside I was feeling sick and anxious, just wanting the time to move quickly and for the baby to be born safely. As well as doing my best to comfort Emma, I touched Sonam's arm and tried to smile. I wanted so desperately to say to both of them that it was 'going to be fine', but I knew I couldn't use those words.

With the blue light flashing and the siren screeching I

struggled to stay upright as we swerved through towns and through traffic lights. It was a desperate situation with Emma pushing hard, and the obstetrician suddenly telling her not to push, as she now wanted to wait until Emma arrived at the hospital. But it was too late and Emma's contractions were expulsive. Grimacing from the pain, she looked at me for reassurance.

'Just do what your body is telling you to do,' I told her.

As we pulled up in the grounds of the hospital the baby's head was visible, and with every second counting we got the stretcher out of the ambulance and raced to the delivery room where Emma immediately gave birth to a baby girl she would name Rose. She was beautiful and cried a little but I was afraid of the consequences of her low heart rate and delayed birth.

'I'm sorry but we have to take her to the neonatal intensive care unit,' the paediatrician, Dr Taylor, told her distressed parents.

Sonam went to the NICU with Rose and I stayed with Emma while she had her stitches. Then I escorted Emma there too.

The medical team met with Emma and Sonam to tell them that Rose was very sick, and that she could have suffered permanent damage. Both parents were naturally in shock, bewildered and worried about what the future would hold.

'If I'd been in hospital would this have happened?' Emma asked me, when she was back in her room.

I didn't have the answer but explained to Emma that similar events had happened in hospital.

'Even with medical assistance on hand the baby can sometimes be compromised,' I told her gently. 'Even the slightest delay can cause problems. Having your baby in hospital does not assure a problem-free birth.'

We both cried, and talked more.

That night I couldn't sleep. I went through every minute of Emma's labour to try to think if there was any earlier indication of Rose's distress. I did feel that everything was in order and that I had been vigilant and thorough.

Whenever a baby was born with complications or problems it is standard procedure for a senior midwife to examine the case records to check that care was appropriate, so I wasn't surprised to be called in the next day to see my manager Miss Harris and my supervisor, Jenny.

When I arrived at the office they were both sat down waiting for me.

'How are you, Sheena?' Jenny asked.

The softness in her voice immediately set me off. Voice wobbling, I explained that I was feeling very distressed as I'd been supporting Emma ever since the birth and hadn't slept.

They assured me that they had spent time reading my records and that all the care I'd given was good and that there were no issues.

'It is obviously a very difficult situation,' Jenny sympathised.

I left not necessarily feeling better but at least assured that my records reflected the good care I knew I had given. I didn't feel the same support from some of my colleagues, however, who either didn't mention the event, or made comments about the appropriateness of home births.

'Well, she shouldn't have had her baby at home,' I heard one of the midwives from delivery suite say. No doubt I was being hypersensitive but it almost felt like they were blaming me. Reading between the lines it seemed they thought I should have encouraged Emma to have her baby in hospital.

There is still a divide between midwives as to whether they support a woman's choice regarding the place of birth. Some midwives have witnessed the amazing experience of caring for a woman at home during labour and birth, and others have only practised in a hospital setting, and feel anxious about the lack of medical assistance. But if women have no current or expected complications and are supported by confident, skilled midwives, the evidence is clear that home birth is as safe as hospital birth. I have never really recovered from the rare events surrounding Rose's birth, but truly believe that women have the right to choose where their baby is born, and that a hospital birth isn't necessarily the safest option.

When an unexpected incident arises today, midwives generally gather round their colleague to offer support, and it makes an enormous difference in helping you to pick yourself up and carry on. Following Rose's birth I didn't feel supported, except from the one meeting with my superiors. It was such a shame.

As I had feared, the next few days were filled with distressing news: Rose had severe cerebral palsy and needed round-the-clock care. I felt terrible for Emma and played the birth over and over in my mind, wondering if there was anything that could have been done differently. The outcome was just so bleak and it made me feel numb.

It was three weeks before Emma was able to take Rose home but she and Sonam faced an exhausting time ahead.

They were plunged into a life of despair and extreme tiredness as Rose screamed around the clock and could not be put down even for a second. They had huge battles trying to get the most appropriate care for her. Although there was little I could do or say I really wanted to help the family so I stayed in touch for a long time.

Meanwhile my children were growing up fast and Anna, my eldest daughter, was soon about to turn nineteen.

When her school days had come to an end Anna had decided to take a gap year to travel before starting university to do a media studies degree. While she was waiting to start she came to our hospital to take part in an educational film about midwives that was being produced by the region's Chief Supervisor of Midwives, Marian Drazec. Marian was producing a film for midwives about the importance of supervision of midwifery and needed a few 'extras', so seeing as Anna was home for a few days I asked if she'd like to help out. Anna was given the role of the mother of a baby who was in the NICU and she really enjoyed getting into the part.

Anna had never really been interested in my work before, but this small insight into hospital life had clearly given her food for thought.

'Mum, I'm thinking of changing my course,' she confided, to my astonishment. 'I would like to look into becoming a midwife!'

She added that she felt that midwifery would be a more meaningful career for her than what she was planning, and that she would be in a position to make a real difference in people's lives.

I was very surprised, and thought it was probably a flash in the pan and that Anna would change her mind again. But she didn't! Anna investigated the potential to apply to study midwifery and chose Birmingham, as she was currently living there with her boyfriend, Shaun.

It all happened so quickly, but Anna applied and was successful. It was the start of what was going to be an amazing experience for me – watching as Anna learned the same profession. In years to come we would drive our family mad as we shared our ideas and knowledge and debated philosophies about midwifery.

My work in the community continued, then in 1997 I decided to apply to become a supervisor of midwives – a role that involved supporting other midwives in their practice to ensure safe care for mothers and babies.

By becoming a supervisor I would be able to lead a team of midwives and help them to improve our service. I really fancied the challenge. There was a selection process and a specialist education programme prior to my successful appointment.

Meanwhile the way my colleagues and I provided care was to change radically. About a year and a half after I first started in the community, the plans Mrs Quinn had been diligently working on finally came to fruition.

'Team midwifery' was introduced – a new system in

which women who had straightforward pregnancies and were expected to have normal births would be cared for by a team of midwives and wouldn't need to see a doctor. This is called midwife-led care.

The midwives would provide twenty-four-hour cover for a number of women, providing them with support all the way through pregnancy, labour and the postnatal period.

The old system of separate community and hospital midwives was being phased out, to be replaced by a new model in which a team of midwives would provide care in and out of the hospital.

It also meant a job change for me and a good deal more responsibility. Mrs Quinn and my manager (a lady called Jenny) asked if I would move from my rural area in the Ribble Valley to be team leader of an urban district in Blackburn. There I would be managing a group of midwives based within the hospital. It would also mean a return to shift work – lates, earlies and nights – once more. It was not a prospect that I relished, but team midwifery was something I really believed in so I was determined to grasp this new opportunity.

The community I was now working in could not have been more different to the affluent and rural Ribble Valley. Blackburn is an old mill town, and following its post-industrial decline in prosperity, it has several pockets of deprivation. There were high levels of unemployment and all the associated social problems that come with that. Blackburn was also culturally diverse, with a high number of south Asian heritage communities. In fact, the Muslim population in Blackburn is one of the highest among all local authorities in the United Kingdom and the highest outside London.

Individuals moved to Lancashire from India and Pakistan in the 1950s for better opportunities and improved lifestyles, and families and friends followed. These families tend to live in defined communities, preferring to live near kinfolk, so these areas of Blackburn often resembled their native countries. I loved working with women and families from these communities and learned so much from them, especially the women.

I was always made welcome when I went to visit mothers and babies after the birth with copious amounts of 'milky' tea and platefuls of Indian delicacies. Soon my enjoyment of their food was showing on the weighing scales!

I made so many friends and used to be invited regularly for meals in their homes. They taught me a huge amount about their culture, their religion, their traditions and how to cook Indian and Pakistani food.

However, it took me a while to get used to my new patch and on a few occasions I did get lost while out on my community visits. When you add the language barriers into the mix it is easy to see how occasionally I got in a bit of a muddle.

Although from time to time we'd have an interpreter available, often I'd do my best to explain why I was visiting in simple English. During one of my first postnatal visits, after grappling with my map for some time, I arrived at the door of a terraced house to be met by an Asian gentleman.

'Hi, I am the midwife,' I said, introducing myself. 'My name is Sheena, can I come in please?'

'Come in. Wife out. Coming back,' he told me, with a smile.

Stepping inside I sat on the settee and spent an awkward fifteen minutes (it felt more like an hour) smiling politely at this man, as we couldn't really have a conversation. He was slightly agitated and kept looking at his watch.

'She coming,' he assured me.

Finally his wife came rushing in with several bags of shopping. I was surprised to see her out and about so soon after the birth, as usually Muslim women don't go outside for forty days. Also, there was no baby! But then Grandma could be minding him, I thought.

'Where's the baby?' I asked with a smile.

'The baby is at school!' she replied.

It was only then that I realised I'd got the wrong house. They must have thought I was a health visitor. I explained myself – well, as best I could – and left shame-faced in pursuit of the right house. Ugh.

This wasn't my only cultural problem. While my task of introducing midwifery-led care and the 'team' approach was generally straightforward with English women, at first I found that women from south Asian backgrounds were skeptical.

'But we want to see the doctor at the hospital!' they said. My colleague Mustary, who was a language-link worker, told me the reason why.

'At home [in India or Pakistan] the doctor is the one with status,' she explained. 'If you see the midwife instead of the doctor it means you can't afford the doctor and so you would feel ashamed.'

So Mustary, Tuhina and Aysha helped us to get the message across that in England the midwives were very experienced and capable of seeing women who don't have problems throughout their whole childbirth experience. Plus there was the big advantage of not having to go to hospital and wait for hours in queues!

To our delight, within two years the women from these communities were asking for midwifery-led care and those who had already had it were asking for 'their team' when they had second or third pregnancies.

Busy days were the norm for team midwifery and certainly the new way of working meant long working hours and more pressure when faced with some of the complex social problems.

Working in a deprived area I saw extreme poverty. It's hard to imagine the degree of desperation experienced by some of the individuals I cared for and difficult to believe that the conditions they lived in even exist in the UK.

I also witnessed the associated ill health that comes with limited access to information and health care. There were women living in isolation and fear and seemingly unable to help themselves, due to poor parenting and life skills, lack of available finances and poor education.

I met women who misused drugs and drank large amounts of alcohol during pregnancy, women trapped in abusive relationships and women suffering from mental health problems.

I was struck by the potential of midwives to help them – yet also our inadequacy. As midwives we were with women at a very important period in their lives and at a time when women were most likely to be susceptible to change. In an ideal world the right approach could be used to support mothers to make lifestyle changes that may help them and their baby to be as healthy as possible. But in reality we were already pushed for time and understandably sometimes midwives felt unable to help with more complex issues. More importantly, we were frequently unaware of other agencies that were able to support women and families. However, there was a shift to consider our greater social responsibility and the potential we had to make a difference.

Some of the women I met were amazing. They dealt with the daily grind of their lives so courageously. With what seemed like a world of troubles on their shoulders they held families together, utilising their inner strength and battling on. Others had hidden talents just waiting to be released and I was to learn very soon how midwives and a positive childbirth experience could be the link to women 'starting over' or having a new lease of life.

One of the GPs I worked for in Blackburn had a surgery in a very run-down area of town where many terraced houses were empty and boarded up.

The surgery itself was in a former house and in quite a state of disrepair. When you stepped inside there was a waiting area to the right, a small dingy room with a gas fire on the wall and six chairs arranged around a battered old coffee table. It was so small that if one patient coughed in the room, the rest would surely be infected.

Facing the front door was a narrow, steep staircase, covered with linoleum that was peeling up at the corners and worn out. Pregnant women had to go upstairs for their antenatal check and I was always worried about them slipping or falling on the lino. Eventually I mentioned my concerns to the receptionist.

'Oh, he won't do anything about it,' she replied in a hostile manner. 'He's too busy.' When I then spoke to the doctor himself he told me it was in hand, and that workmen would be arriving shortly to replace the flooring. But it never happened.

The equipment in the upstairs room where we held the antenatal clinic was also old and broken, but luckily anything that we needed to use we brought ourselves.

It was at this clinic that I first became aware of the increasing number of teenagers who were pregnant. Girls as young as fifteen were attending antenatal clinics, coming with their friends and having little or no input from a mother figure or family member.

I would try to talk to them and encourage them to join in some of the antenatal (parentcraft) sessions that were being held in the community or at the hospital.

'No thanks,' was the usual mumbled reply. 'I'll feel embarrassed.'

Most of the girls said they would feel out of place with 'older' women, and some didn't have partners and didn't want the fact that they were single to be highlighted. Others just sat quietly saying nothing but never arrived at the parentcraft sessions.

When I asked the other members of my team if they were noticing more teenage girls in certain areas, they agreed they had noticed an increase.

I felt frustrated. On the whole I found the girls I met

were interested in information about labour, birth and childcare. They just needed a chance, and the right approach, but during the busy clinic sessions I didn't have time to spend with them. I really didn't feel teenagers were getting the right support and as a potentially vulnerable group they were unprepared for birth and a new baby.

I spoke to my manager about my concerns, and although she acknowledged the problem, there weren't any extra resources available to change the situation, so we carried on much the same.

Although I was now working in Blackburn I was still in touch with Emma, Sonam and Rose, and often visited their home in Clitheroe.

I loved the family, and enjoyed their company. It was still a huge struggle for Emma and Sonam to get the right support for Rose and they were constantly exhausted.

But now they had happy news. Emma was pregnant again with her second child and I was touched to hear that she had written to Mrs Quinn to ask if special permission could be given for me to be her midwife for the birth.

I was overwhelmed when I read a copy of that letter. Emma trusted me. I was going to be her midwife again and I was so grateful.

Although Emma wanted another home birth it was eventually agreed she would give birth in hospital because of a low-lying placenta, and luckily I was available to be her midwife once more. Thankfully this time Emma's labour was fine and her daughter Jessica was born with no complications or problems.

The friendship between our two families grew, until one day Emma invited me to her house. After we'd caught up on each other's news she revealed that she was thinking of instigating a claim against the hospital for negligence during Rose's birth.

She told me that she had been at a friend's garden party and heard a solicitor talking about birth injury. Emma had chatted to him afterwards and they briefly discussed Rose. The solicitor had encouraged Emma to let him look into the events surrounding Rose's birth.

'What do you think?' she asked me. 'We obviously don't want you to be upset and we know you gave us good care, but we also want to investigate other things, such as the delay with the ambulance.'

I knew that Emma and Sonam were still finding life hard with intense twenty-four-hour a day care needed for Rose. Support continued to be minimal and they had to fight tooth and nail for the little they had. The family was weary and emotional and had not been given the chance to come to terms with the enormity of what had happened. No counselling had been offered, and there had been no support in assimilating this experience and no chance to discuss it. Whilst the potential for financial support to help with Rose's care was a strong reason for them to go ahead, Emma and Sonam were also desperate to make sense of their experience. They suspected that there had been mistakes made but had never had the opportunity to investigate. Now through litigation they could get those much-needed explanations.

I didn't know what to say. I was totally surprised by

the decision but I understood their despair. I hadn't ever been in this position before, so really didn't know what to think. I was fairly naïve and concluded that if Emma did proceed then it wouldn't affect me. After all, none of it was my fault.

'You have to do what you think is right, Emma,' I told her. 'It's really up to you.'

The following day I went to discuss the conversation with my manager, who explained briefly what would happen if Emma's litigation plan went ahead. Again, I wasn't overly worried.

A period of time passed and duly the Trust received a letter to say Emma was claiming for damages. Her solicitor had asked for statements from everyone involved. Suddenly I was warned there was going to be a lot of input from me as I'd given most of the care.

When I saw the first statements I was terribly shocked. There were things written that didn't chime with my memory of events. Before long I would learn that this situation would arise time and time again and the process I had entered would be a continuous stream of statements and responses.

I was instructed not to have contact with Emma and her family, which was sad and frustrating. As I pored over the paperwork I couldn't ask her why things had been written, or, after reading a strongly worded paragraph about my care, I couldn't pick up the phone to explain to her why I had responded in a certain way.

It was dreadful. Emma was my friend, and yet we were being driven apart. As it turned out the litigation process was to last for many years and would consist of meetings with solicitors, barristers, supervisors of midwives, Royal College of Midwives representatives and more.

The activity came in bursts. Sometimes a year would go by, and I wouldn't hear anything, then out of the blue, wham. It was back again. Time and again Jane, the solicitor allocated to represent the Trust, would talk me through another damning statement.

At first the focus was on the ambulance delay and all the details surrounding that. Then the big blow came. As my colleague Linda and I sat in an austere barristers' chambers in London we were informed that causation of Rose's brain injury couldn't be associated with the delay in the ambulance. Even if the ambulance had arrived on time the baby would have been compromised.

With that angle for litigation closed the claimants' solicitors were turning their attention to my care.

I was completely shocked and devastated. How could I now be blamed?

There were more statements, more meetings and more tears.

I often thought about Emma and her family and felt both touched and sad when Christmas cards arrived from them. Despite all the stress I understood Emma's heartache and still wished I could have helped her more.

Chapter 12

Sat in a boardroom I looked round at the sea of faces as one by one they introduced themselves. Everyone looked so important and I suddenly felt overawed and intimidated.

'Um, my name is Sheena Byrom,' I managed to stammer when it was my turn. 'And I'm a midwifery team leader in Blackburn.'

I could hardly believe that here I was on a Primary Care Group Board. It was all very surreal.

The position had come about after I was asked by my manager if I'd consider putting my name forward. I'd jumped at the chance.

Primary Care Groups (or PCGs) were made up of local GPs, nurses, social service representatives and various other personnel and had been established in an attempt by the Department of Health to modernise the NHS in the UK.

I knew that PCGs would be responsible for ensuring health inequalities were addressed in socio-economically deprived areas, so this opportunity could bring me a chance to really make a difference.

My manager explained that as they needed two 'nurse' representatives (which in the small print included midwives) to be on the board it would be good for some midwives to put their names forward.

There was quite a lot of work involved. I had to develop a manifesto outlining why and how I would be able to help with the development of a new local service, which would be circulated to all community-based nurses, midwives and health visitors. With all these health workers voting for candidates they liked most I knew I'd have to word it just right to get my point across. It took me hours to complete.

Well, my hard work paid off and I was thrilled to discover that I'd been elected for the Blackburn with Darwen Board. I was very pleased but also scared. What had I done? I arrived at the first meeting feeling pretty nervous.

After all the introductions had been completed we talked about the role of the group and the sort of projects we could be supporting. It may have been nerve-wracking at first but I found it very interesting.

However, if I thought interacting with my fellow board members was scary, the nurses were something else.

Every month it was the job of Vera, the other nursing representative, and myself to update groups of nurses in the community with progress from the board. This took place at GP practices where we would address groups of ten.

I quickly noticed that while they were happy to listen to Vera, some of the women were unhappy with the fact that a midwife had been elected and not a nurse (although I had been a nurse too!). And some of them could be quite rude.

'You won't understand this because you're a midwife,' was a common put-down.

However, I think this experience made me stronger. I

learned to challenge appropriately and calmly and to listen and accept that I couldn't always make things better.

Being on the board also undoubtedly helped me to have a greater understanding of the politics associated with health care. I witnessed the flaws of important decision-making and how the personalities of a strategic group could influence major local health service changes.

It was quite a challenge doing this work on top of my role as a midwifery team leader. Commitments sometimes clashed and I had to prioritise without letting my colleagues down. Sometimes I would be sat in an important meeting in the morning and back on the delivery suite catching babies in the afternoon!

The real sense of achievement came from the potential to make a difference. I was often first to hear about initiatives that could help to improve maternity services and a great opportunity soon arose at one of the meetings.

It was at a meeting of a subcommittee of the board, which had been established to address the high levels of coronary heart disease (CHD) in the area. During the meeting it was revealed that there were financial resources for projects that help to reduce CHD.

After passing on the information about the opportunity to the various nurses working within the community in Blackburn I went to speak to my midwifery colleagues about how we could access some of the funding.

'But we can't reduce coronary heart disease!' one senior midwife proclaimed. 'We are midwives!'

I went home and tossed and turned in bed that night, wracking my brain. Then at about 3 a.m. a thought suddenly came to me. I was sure I could recall reading something about low birth weight and heart disease.

For the next two days I did some research and phoned my cousin, Barbara, for a chat. Barbara Swan OBE was my Aunt Maud's second daughter and at the time worked as a clinical manager in community nursing in Stockport. Her role focused on public health approaches to health care, which meant that with her team she developed innovative ways to help improve the health of those communities most in need.

Instead of using a 'top-down' approach where health professionals know best and 'teach' the patient, the philosophy of public health work is to try to engage with communities at their level and on their terms, and to 'share not own' information.

The aim of this approach is to reduce the great paradox of health care – the fact that those who are most in need of medical care are the least likely people to receive it.

'I'm sure there is something we can do here,' I told Barbara, revealing the research I'd found (the 'Barker Hypothesis') that demonstrated how babies born with a low birth weight due to poor growth in the uterus were more likely to have heart disease in later life. Barbara knew about this and sent me more information.

As we chatted I remembered the teenagers I'd met in deprived parts of Blackburn and how they needed more support. There was also some research that teenagers had smaller babies . . . That was it! I could apply for some funding to run a specific project for pregnant teenagers to try to support them to have a healthy-sized baby – with the outcome of reducing heart disease in the future!

It was a long shot, but I really wanted to do it. I needed to write up the idea for the fund holder and the proposal would be considered by a panel later in the month.

I had never written a proposal before, so Barbara agreed to help me and for several weeks we conversed back and forth via email until finally it was ready.

My big concern was that it wasn't going to impress the panel, as they were looking for projects where the results would be immediate.

But almost two weeks later the news came that it had been accepted and I was given the go-ahead to start with the planning. I couldn't wait to get back to base to tell the others. It was *so* exciting!

This now meant that we could develop a plan to have a midwife specifically dealing with teenage pregnancy. The post we created was one of the first in the country and we developed a second post with other external funding a few years later. The impact of having a teenage pregnancy midwife was almost immediate and in many parts of England similar posts were developed to help address the needs of this vulnerable group.

One of our teenage pregnancy midwives, Lesley, has clearly had an incalculable impact and has established thriving support groups for these young women. The midwives on the delivery suite regularly say they can spot one of Lesley's teenagers a mile off, as they are always 'so well prepared and confident'.

On one occasion Lesley even inspired an eighteen-year-old mother to apply to be a midwife herself. After chatting with Lesley, Sophie, mother to a healthy baby boy, was adamant she was going to be a successful breastfeeder, and on Lesley's advice joined a teenage pregnancy support group where she could get further help with feeding, pregnancy, parenting and further education.

Sophie attended the group every week and continued breastfeeding for many months. The group enabled Sophie to get the weekly support she needed not only for the continuation of breastfeeding but in all aspects of the care of her newborn – as well as giving her the chance to meet new friends. Sophie would come to the group and breastfeed her baby and in doing so she encouraged other teenagers to breastfeed their tiny charges too.

Eventually Sophie decided she would like to become a midwife herself. She enrolled in a college course with a view to eventually becoming a midwife and recently completed a breastfeeding course within the hospital so that she could train to be a volunteer support worker with other breast-feeding mothers. It was a real testament to the good work Lesley and her colleagues carry out on a weekly basis.

As for me, in 2000, after three years working as a team leader, I was promoted to be a community midwife manager. This was quite a culture shock for me as it meant I would potentially be delivering far fewer babies myself. Now, rather than supporting mothers giving birth, I was supporting the midwives who were supporting the mothers.

At first I didn't feel particularly happy in my new role. I had much less job satisfaction, and I wasn't sure it was for me. I missed the close contact with women and families and felt like there was a huge void in my work life.

Now I was hearing all about midwives and the difficult hurdles they faced, and I realised a lot of careful consideration would be needed to work out how best to proceed in some cases. Their concerns could be in relation to their home life, or work patterns, or the fact that there was a staffing shortage. Sometimes the problem would be about a family they were caring for that they weren't sure how to deal with.

My approach followed the one I had with the mothers – listening, talking and attempting to help them to find a solution themselves. I noticed that when I worked in this way, encouraging, empowering and supporting when difficulties emerged, midwives and other members of staff responded well.

When I received positive feedback from a colleague my confidence returned, and I started to enjoy the leadership role. Six months in I was definitely much more inspired and determined to succeed in my new position. I realised I just needed to be a midwife to the midwives.

One winter afternoon I was sat at my desk when Sam, one of the midwives I managed, called in a distressed state about a woman she'd seen in her antenatal clinic that morning.

She said she'd been examining a woman, who was thirty-four weeks' pregnant, when she'd discovered that the foetus was in a breech position. When Sam explained this to the woman she suddenly became very aggressive.

'That's it,' she said, pushing my colleague away and getting down from the examination couch. 'I'm not coming back. I'm going home.'

Sam was upset about the way she'd been spoken to but also because the woman, Dawn, had said she didn't want any further antenatal care. Sam was at a loss as to what to do.

After reassuring Sam I called Dawn at home to see if I could find out what the problem was and was immediately met with a torrent of abuse.

'How dare you ring my house!' she shouted. 'How dare you interfere! I'm going to have my baby on my own. I don't need you, you are all stupid.'

Then she hung up. I was really taken aback.

Unsure how to proceed, I went to see my manager, Mrs Quinn.

'She seems adamant that we shouldn't be involved but we need to make sure she's safe,' I explained.

'You need to get in touch with her again,' Mrs Quinn told me firmly. 'Either ring her again or write to her, she obviously needs support.'

So the next day I plucked up the courage and called Dawn again, this time determined to use a different tactic. As soon as she answered the phone I quickly told her that I was sorry she was so upset and that because there was a problem I'd like to come and meet her.

'Who do you think you are?' she began, her voice oozing with hostility.

'Please, if I come I won't speak,' I quickly interrupted. 'I'll sit and listen.'

There was a pause while she thought about it.

'OK, you can come,' she shouted. 'But if you dare to open your mouth you'll be dead.'

Arriving at her address the next day I have to admit I felt very anxious. I didn't know what to expect, but I did know that my approach needed to be gentle and submissive.

When I rang the doorbell the woman, Dawn, opened the door and loomed over me from a higher step. She seemed taller than me too, and had an angry, troubled face.

'Hi, I'm Sheena,' I said quietly, smiling at her.

'You can come in,' she said, jabbing her finger in my face. 'But don't speak.'

I followed her inside and she instructed me where to sit. She then launched into an angry rant about how horrendous our maternity service was. She said she had two children already and her care had been terrible. Her second baby had been in a breech position and the doctor had 'made her' have a Caesarean section.

'There was no choice,' she exclaimed, her voice filled with agitation. 'He just came in with another male doctor and told me I had to go to theatre. I was petrified.' Dawn then told me how she found out the day after the section that she may not have needed the operation and that as it was her second baby, she should have been offered the choice of having the baby vaginally.

'Afterwards I couldn't look after my first child,' she said. 'I felt like I'd had no say in the matter and I felt totally abused.'

She added that in the past she'd had abusive relationships and it just felt like yet another occasion where a man had taken control of her.

'You can do what you like, but I'm not coming into

hospital to have another man mistreat me,' she told me defensively.

Suddenly I didn't feel anxious or scared any more. I just felt sad for her. I realised Dawn was asserting her authority because she'd been badly let down. I sat and listened as she continued.

'What do you think?' she eventually said.

'Would you like me to speak?' I asked. She pursed her lips and nodded but avoided eye contact.

'Well, at this stage I just feel sorry that you've had such a terrible ordeal,' I said softly. 'Maybe I could come another day and see how I can support you?'

She put her head down and thought about it.

'OK, you can come next Tuesday,' she agreed.

As I went to leave, I noticed there seemed to be something else bothering her.

'Can you check my baby is OK?' she eventually asked.

So I got my equipment from the car and she lay down on the sofa so I could examine her. I checked the baby's heartbeat and told her gently that the baby was still breech.

When I returned the following week she still seemed a little angry but was less aggressive. She told me again how unhappy she was and when she'd finished I once more asked if it was OK for me to speak. She nodded.

'What would you like to do?' I asked. 'What is the best way we can help you?'

'I'm not coming to hospital,' she told me adamantly. 'I am going to have this baby here, on my own.'

I carefully and sensitively explained that it would be

unsafe to have her baby without help, and would potentially put her and her baby at risk.

'Perhaps we could send a midwife to you?' I ventured. Another long pause.

'Yes,' she replied. 'But I want to meet her first.'

I explained that I would speak to my colleagues and to the midwives, and that we would have to make a careful plan.

'If there was a problem would you come in to hospital?' I asked.

'If the baby could die, then yes,' she agreed. I promised to get back to her the following day with some more information and as she saw me to the door I noticed she was now looking me in the eye.

'Thank you for everything,' she said. Then she stood on the doorstep and waved me off, smiling. The experience made me feel sad and humble. Behind all the aggression and bravado was a woman who simply wanted to be listened to.

Back at the hospital I talked to my colleagues and two midwives came forward and said they'd like to support her. I arranged for them to liaise with Dawn over the next week and they provided all her care from then on.

Dawn was happy with this, and also agreed to the plan that if the baby was still breech when she went into labour an ambulance would be stationed outside, ready to transfer her in to the hospital if necessary. The midwives were given extra training on breech birth and were supported by managers and supervisors of midwives at every stage.

As it happened, Dawn's baby turned round and was born head-first at home, two days after her due date. She had a wonderful experience and when I called her a week later to see how things were, she was happy and said it was the best birth she'd ever had.

'Thank you for everything,' she said. 'I'll never forget you and the midwives and the support they gave me.'

I sat back after the call and thought about how little it takes to really support women. The focus should always be on the individual, her circumstances, her feelings and her ability to communicate them.

But it was not always easy. As well as dealing with vulnerable women like Dawn, I was becoming increasingly aware of the challenges of supporting women with addictions, especially drug and alcohol dependence.

The midwives in my team often felt they were failing women who struggled to cope with everyday life due to drug misuse. They reported that the women seemed 'lost', usually not attending routine check-ups or avoiding contact with health services for many reasons. Some of the midwives found it hard, as I had done in their position, and came to me with extraordinary stories for support and reassurance.

Shauna, one of the team midwives, reported going to check on a nineteen-year-old girl with a longstanding drugs problem who was expecting her first baby. Shauna was worried as Rosa hadn't been coming to her antenatal checks and hadn't been at home when she'd visited.

Weeks went by without Rosa having any sort of check-up but eventually, after some probing, Shauna found a new address for Rosa and managed to catch her when she called in just after teatime.

Rosa needed a blood test to check her iron levels and

Shauna could never have imagined the scene that unravelled next.

As Shauna knelt on the floor next to Rosa's seat having just inserted the needle into her arm, the door was propelled off its hinges as the police burst in. They were looking for drugs and for Rosa's partner in relation to drugs offences (he escaped out of the back bedroom window but was subsequently caught and ended up in prison).

It was quite a scene, but Shauna, ever the professional, took it all in her stride, finishing the task at hand before ensuring Rosa had what she needed and calmly packing up and leaving. She did wonder afterwards if, at first glance, the police had thought that she too was part of the drugs scene. From then on Shauna was in close contact with Rosa, and she built up a close bond. Sadly, however, Rosa's baby boy needed intensive medical care immediately after birth and it took weeks before he was allowed home to the foster parents that social services had found for him.

Being placed in foster care was not an unusual outcome for babies born to women with drug dependencies. In fact, one of the reasons that women avoided health services in pregnancy was that they feared they might have their baby removed into care.

Seeing as there was no specialist midwifery service for pregnant women who used drugs, women with this problem would frequently not come for help until late in their pregnancy or they were in labour.

This meant that often the baby would be affected and would have to be admitted to the neonatal intensive care unit (NICU), like Rosa's baby, for observation and treatment.

If the mother had not attended for antenatal care, social services would only be contacted at this point, meaning that there would be no pre-birth assessment of the home situation. As a result, emergency decisions were often made to the detriment of the mother and father, resulting in the baby being removed unnecessarily from the family.

This was something that the other community midwifery manager, Janice, and I were keen to tackle. So together we set up meetings with the drug and alcohol service in Blackburn to see if there was any way we could improve care for pregnant women who were using these substances.

There was a full agreement that the service was needed and after writing a lengthy 'bid' for extra funding we were delighted to discover the drugs service was willing to part-fund a specialist drug midwife post.

This was a momentous step forward. It meant that when a woman who used drugs or alcohol became pregnant she would immediately be referred for extra support. The specialist midwife would have knowledge on the problems encountered by these women, and how best to care for the woman and her family. It didn't take long for the post to have an impact although the job was at times gruelling for our specialist midwife, Joanne.

Often Joanne would come to speak to Janice and me about the women for whom she was caring. Sometimes she would be working in extremely difficult, distressing and emotionally draining circumstances.

She relayed one story about a woman called Jody who had recently been released from prison, as had her partner, Tommy.

They had both spent a number of years in foster care and children's homes and were both addicted to drugs. Jody was using crack cocaine and heroin and Tommy was using heroin, and they had done so since their teenage years.

They'd already had a baby girl who was seven months old. She'd been removed shortly after birth and was now adopted. The distress was so intense when the baby was removed that in order to cope with their feelings of grief and loss, their drug use increased. The couple were living in a bus shelter in Accrington at night and walking the streets by day.

When Jody realised she was pregnant again she was happy but worried. It was winter and so very cold and they were spending all their money on heroin and crack cocaine.

Eventually Jody resorted to prostitution to earn the £100- to £200-worth of heroin and crack they used each day. At first they didn't tell social services about the pregnancy but eventually Jody told a worker in the needle exchange. She was given a pregnancy test and referred on to the specialist midwife, Joanne.

Initially Jody was rude to Joanne. She wouldn't give her eye contact or engage at all. She was unsure about being referred to the substance misuse team, where Tommy was already in treatment and being prescribed methadone, as she thought that this would make her look like a 'bad mother'.

'I'm not having my baby taken away again,' she snapped at Joanne.

But eventually Jody relented and agreed to be seen. As with Tommy, they prescribed methadone, a synthetic opiate-based medicine, which is used to stop the symptoms of withdrawal.

With the help of a key worker Jody gradually gave up the drug abuse (as did Tommy) and she stopped the prostitution.

Eventually the social care team became involved and a plan of support was arranged. The couple found out the sex of the baby and started to bond with him. Jody went into labour on her due date and gave birth to her baby boy. Joanne, together with the drugs team and social services, managed to get funding for supported accommodation in a family rehabilitation unit, so that the family could stay together and receive intensive support.

Six months later Joanne heard that Jody, Tommy and the baby were doing exceptionally well, and were now living in a rented house in a better area. It was a hugely encouraging result.

Joanne used to tell me that whilst the work she did was sometimes stressful, she felt very fortunate in doing a job she enjoyed. 'The majority of women use drugs or alcohol as self-medication to shut out things that are too painful to bear, like bereavement or abuse,' she told me. 'I like it that I can help.'

There is still a midwife working in this role today and her work has been invaluable in reducing the admission of babies to the NICU. Working with the substance misuse teams, supporting women and enabling them to make choices around their substance use has also contributed to a reduction in the number of babies being removed from their parents after birth, which is wonderful to know.

*

Every day as a manager would bring something new. As well as unburdening themselves of their problems, mid-wives would also come to me to report memorable births, mostly wonderfully heartwarming but some with strange or bizarre outcomes.

One senior midwife, Laura, came to tell me about a home birth she'd attended the day before. The baby had been born normally but as she was trying to deliver the placenta, the cord had snapped off and couldn't be seen in the vagina. This sometimes happens, but is usually followed by the placenta appearing shortly afterwards.

'I tried all sorts,' Laura confided. 'But then when the mother said she needed to pee I thought that would do the trick.'

Laura thought that the placenta would come once the woman's bladder was empty and that the pressure of sitting on the loo would certainly help move things along.

But on her return from the toilet the woman was shaking her head and Laura and her colleague were disappointed when after another ten minutes the placenta was still nowhere to be seen.

Laura was just about to ring the hospital to arrange transfer in, when Susan, her midwife colleague, went to use the loo herself.

'There it was in the bottom of the toilet, all intact!' Laura exclaimed.

How the woman had failed to see it was a mystery but she was very relieved to stay at home and cuddle up with her baby.

*

Meanwhile the subject of Emma's birth and the ongoing litigation case never lost momentum over the years but one day, in March 2002, it took an upsetting new twist.

I was walking back to my office after a long and stressful meeting when Angela, one of my colleagues, approached me in the corridor.

'Sheena, I need to speak to you,' she said. She followed me into my office and closed the door.

'I think you need to see this,' she said, handing me the local paper.

'BLIND GIRL IN COURT BATTLE – six-year-old sues hospital bosses,' the headline read. It was related to Emma's legal case.

Scanning the article I realised with horror that not only was my name there, in black and white, but it went on to list a series of alleged failings on my part during the care of Emma in labour.

The allegations that were in the press were the opinion of an expert witness employed by Emma's solicitor. It was routine for each 'side' to obtain expert advice from relevant professionals – in this case midwives and obstetricians. Both the claimant (Emma) and the defendant (the hospital I worked for) had expert witnesses whose views on my practice varied greatly. I had seen these allegations when I'd attended the meeting in London and they'd made uneasy reading. What had alarmed me the most was that the expert finding fault in my practice was a senior employee at the Royal College of Midwives.

The role of the College includes setting and supporting standards for midwifery practice from a professional perspective and lobbying the government for better pay or working conditions for midwives. From the legal team's perspective this meant that the comments made by an employee of the College were more likely to be highly regarded. Yet I'd been reassured that they would not stand up. Never for one minute had I imagined they'd end up on the front page of a newspaper.

Sitting down, I read it again. I felt utterly sick. I believed without doubt that my care for Emma had not contributed to Rose's condition. Yet these allegations had been printed in the paper despite the fact that nothing had been proved. I was totally and utterly devastated.

I rang Paul but could hardly get my words out. Then I immediately went to find my manager, Mrs Quinn. I would have to leave, I thought. I couldn't be a midwife now. This was too bad. Pauline was horrified, too, and together we went to see the chief executive of the Trust.

He was sympathetic but told us that I couldn't and shouldn't respond to the press. He said that if I felt strongly about it I could seek legal advice, so I contacted the Royal College of Midwives to ask for their support and then I went home.

As I drove home my chest felt tight, like I couldn't breathe, as I thought about the repercussions the article was likely to bring. What would the people in my community think? And all the mothers and families I had lovingly cared for over the years? And it wasn't true! My eyes stung with tears and I could barely see the road. I just needed to be with my family as soon as possible.

True to form they were wonderful, gathering around me as I burst through the door in floods.

'Everyone will be talking about me,' I sobbed. 'They won't know it's not true.'

As if on cue the bell went and there on the doorstep was my friend Julie Walsh, armed with dusters and cleaning products. With a determined look on her face she breezed in and started moving stuff around in the kitchen.

'What *are* you doing?' I asked her, as she started to brush.

'I am cleaning,' she answered. 'You won't need to think of this now and I need to do something practical for you. I am furious.'

There were no tears, hugs or kisses: Julie just scrubbed and polished, cleaned my house from top to bottom and then left. Julie has the most amazing knack of knowing how to make people feel better without making a fuss, and that day I knew that she really cared.

I found out later that Julie was driving through Clitheroe when she noticed a billboard with the story emblazoned across it. She was furious and worried that I might see it, so she screeched to a halt, ran across the road and turned the board round. She then went to all the other newsagents in the town and if they had a board displaying the story she moved the board or turned it round! What a friend!

I was also touched when a neighbour popped by with some flowers and Pauline arrived that night with some more. The phone didn't stop ringing with friends keen to tell me not to worry.

I didn't sleep a wink that night. More than anything I wanted to contact Emma to ask her if she had instigated it. It seemed very unlikely but the case hadn't yet been 'heard', so where had all the information come from?

The following day I dragged myself into work. Pauline called me into her office and we rang the legal team. They explained that earlier that week a court hearing had taken place between both legal teams in London that journalists were allowed to attend. When the allegations were read out at the meeting a reporter had picked up on the story.

My big fear was that most people wouldn't necessarily understand the legal system (I didn't) and would take the allegations made against me as fact. It was the enormous injustice of the situation that upset me the most. I knew I hadn't made any mistakes in Emma's care.

Just when I thought things couldn't get any worse the allegations were repeated in my local paper in Clitheroe, a weekly paper that was highly regarded for focusing on positive news and for being more ethically sound.

My children went to school in Clitheroe and I'd grown up there and had lived there when I was a community midwife.

Olivia even came home from school one evening all upset, as someone at school had said that her mummy had damaged a baby. It was awful.

The tears came again, as did the overwhelming nausea. All my career I had strived to do the right thing, to be strong, to care and to keep mothers and babies at the centre of my decisions and now within a week my reputation was shattered. Although lots of my friends and family wrote to the paper to complain about my treatment, the editor refused to print the letters. Ironically he said it was unethical while the legal proceedings were still ongoing.

I tried to keep positive and to be strong, especially at

work. I knew I had a senior position and needed to lead the staff, but inside I was anxious and crumbling. I couldn't sleep and began to get palpitations, which worried me given my family history. I went to see my GP, who of course knew all about it. Everyone did! I felt people were pointing me out to others, or at least registering who I was.

Then one morning about a week later there was a knock on my door. It was Beth Peterson, one of the mothers I had been a midwife for who lived in Clitheroe.

'This is for you,' she said with a concerned but loving look on her face. She handed me a parcel.

When I opened the package there was a fifty-page petition, with more than 400 names and signatures of local mothers protesting against the paper's decision to print the story. I was so touched and humbled by this gesture.

'The women that have signed all know and respect you, Sheena,' she said. 'They are so angry about this and want you to know you have their support.'

I was moved to tears.

'The problem is the editor won't publish or mention the petition on his letters page,' she went on.

Thanking Beth I told her not to worry, she'd done more than enough already. What she had done was incredible and it really brought me so much comfort during a very dark time.

When I sat down to read the names I was overwhelmed, especially as so many signatures were from women I'd looked after during their pregnancy and postnatally. One of my big worries was that people could liken me to Harold Shipman, who was all over the news at the time. But it seemed at least some of the parents I had cared for didn't believe the paper after all and for a little while I felt better.

Desperate to clear my name in some way I went to see a solicitor in London, arranged and paid for by the Royal College of Midwives. While he was sympathetic and thought I could possibly have a case for a claim against the newspapers he said he couldn't guarantee it and it could actually go the other way. He said it could be traumatic for me too. Everything was so fuddled in my head. I was wasting energy on negative thoughts, and felt so disillusioned. I thought of Emma frequently, wondering what she was making of it all.

Emma, as it happened, was pregnant again, and a few months later I bumped into her in the antenatal clinic at the hospital. It was so hard for both of us. We wanted to hug each other, but we couldn't. We smiled and said 'hello', and it felt sad. After that, Emma wrote a beautiful, heartfelt letter saying that it was never her intention to hurt me.

Years later I discovered that she'd actually been visiting family when the story hit the news-stands. She and Sonam had known nothing of it until confronted by neighbours and friends, accusing them of being 'money grabbing' and damaging my career. How horrific it was for them too. They had also felt like everyone was pointing the finger and talking about them and had been left just as mortified. The way the story had been reported had set us on different sides, and that was not the case at all.

And on top of everything they were still struggling with Rose, caring for her round the clock with little support from social services. Their plight was on a different level to mine.

Chapter 13

As stories went it was a harrowing one.

It concerned the case of a young woman called Tara who had fallen under the spell of a domineering partner – a man twenty years her senior who had previously been convicted for sexual and violent abuse of his children.

Tara was very vulnerable, having grown up in care with a history of abuse herself. She saw living with this man as a way out of her troubled past but of course it actually just intensified her problems.

Over a period of three years Tara gave birth to three children, all of whom were removed by social services. It was deeply distressing for her and also very sad for the midwives caring for her.

Now as a senior midwife and a supervisor of midwives I was regularly involved in advising my team how best to deal with sensitive child protection issues.

The area of child protection had become more intense following high-profile cases such as Victoria Climbie, and midwives were often in the middle of support strategies or child care orders.

While a case like Tara's seemed extreme it was not at all

uncommon or unusual. Social problems seemed to be increasing with each year.

I'd often (and still do) hear comments where parents were condemned for their behaviour, especially if the baby was affected by their actions. However, in my experience, it is rare that people are born bad. There is almost always a reason in their background that leads to their seemingly bad choices.

Taking a child away from a mother is heartbreaking for all concerned, especially as you watch the mother doing all she can to put off the moment when the door opens and social workers arrive to take her baby.

I have seen women desperately breastfeeding in a bid to prolong the time or simply begging for a little bit longer to say goodbye.

While I know there are continuing attempts to try to improve parenting skills and reduce the number of children removed from their parents, I often read about initiatives in other countries where special packages of care have been developed to help to keep children and parents together. There are schemes where support workers move in to help and coach rather than removing the baby from the family. I can't help thinking how much better it would be if we had that option here.

As I carried out my day-to-day tasks, doing my best to problem solve as best I could, I also decided to do something very different – a masters degree!

I'd always wanted to try further education and my cousin Barbara really gave me a boost.

'Do a masters, Sheena,' she encouraged. 'Don't bother with a first degree, you are too old!' Charming!

At the time I didn't have a great formal education. I'd failed my eleven-plus exam – despite attempting to pass it twice. And while I'd left school with only five O levels I'd missed out on finishing my A levels due to my parents' illness. And that was where my education had ended.

Over the years I'd done various modules but applying to undertake a masters degree was a huge step. However, I must have written something right on my application as I was accepted.

Gingerly I reminded Paul that I would now be studying part-time, working late into the night on top of my busy day as a midwifery manager. And, um, this would go on for four years.

'And how much will that cost?' he joked, putting his arm round me with a squeeze. I rolled my eyes.

It was going to be exhausting but luckily I enjoyed learning. In fact, I was halfway through my masters when the opportunity arose to climb the career ladder once more.

The year was 2002 and Tony Blair had given the nursing and midwifery profession a much-needed boost, revealing that he wanted to enhance leadership within the profession and introduce a new role to fulfil that vision. As a result, consultant nurse and midwife positions were introduced throughout the country.

This was a real honour for midwifery, as the title 'consultant' was previously associated with senior doctors. The posts were developed within strictly defined criteria: they all had the same core elements and they were only to be introduced in hospitals where the need for such a role had been identified.

Mrs Quinn and her management team, including me, duly spent some time discussing the possibility of having a consultant midwife position in Blackburn. Consequently Mrs Quinn approached the University of Central Lancashire (UCLan) to ask for joint funding for the post. They agreed.

When the decision was made to go ahead, I spoke to Paul about my interest in applying.

'The focus of the role is public health,' I told him. 'I'd love to be involved.'

With our success in creating new specialist midwife roles for teenage mothers and drug-dependent expectant women, I knew the potential was there to do so much more.

One of the essential criteria for the post was a masters degree so I was extremely grateful to my cousin Barbara for encouraging me to study at that level! I duly applied and was one of five people selected for interview, all the other candidates being external applicants.

This was exciting – but if I thought I'd faced intimidating interviews before I really had no idea what I was getting into now.

This time I would be grilled by a terrifying panel of seven senior health officials, including the head of midwifery, the head of the midwifery school at the university, a consultant obstetrician and other strategic leaders from various midwifery sectors.

I also had to present on a specific topic related to the post, and then answer questions afterwards. It was all extremely nerve-wracking.

After a week of preparation and sleepless nights, the morning of the interview came. My grilling would take place first thing so I got there especially early to set everything up.

But inserting my presentation disk into the computer the unthinkable happened. It wouldn't work.

'No!' I muttered under my breath. I tried again. Nothing. I could feel my stomach knotting with panic.

The interviews were being held in one of the seminar rooms on the delivery suite, so I ran out and grabbed various passing colleagues, pleading with them to help me to get it to work.

Eventually one of the obstetricians, Simon, who was on the interview panel himself, was able to help me get my notes to load on to the computer screen – although not the big projector screen as I had intended. Damn. It would have to do. Thankfully I also had paper handouts of my presentation.

The interview panel certainly put me through my paces.

'How will you develop this new role and what would be your priority?' asked Pauline Quinn.

'I would speak to key members of staff and women who use the service to ascertain what they thought,' I replied.

'How will you develop research capacity within the unit?' an obstetrician fired.

It was mentioned that I hadn't worked in any other unit and I felt that this was frowned upon.

'Why have you not moved to another health authority?' asked the chief supervisor of midwives. 'Do you see the fact you have never moved as a barrier?'

'I haven't been able to move as I have a husband with a good job, four children and a sick mother,' I answered honestly. 'But I see it as an advantage,' I added. 'I know the community we serve so I feel I already have a head start with this job.'

I added that I had a vested interest in the service as my children would be using it.

With my intense hour-and-a-half interview over I left the room feeling pretty flushed and exhausted. Although I hardly dared to hope, I thought it had gone fairly well but there was no doubt I was up against some serious competition. I knew most of the other candidates and they were good.

I'd expected a few sleepless nights while I awaited my fate but later that day I was called into the office by Pauline.

'Congratulations!' she said, beaming from ear to ear.

I wanted to hug her.

It was wonderful to see she was as excited as I was. I held Pauline in high esteem and I was elated.

I immediately called Paul, crying tears of joy, and from the sound of his voice I could tell he was pretty choked too. What an achievement and a huge privilege! I was ecstatically happy as I drove home to my family that night.

Working as a consultant midwife was probably the best job I had in my career and I loved every minute of it.

My post entailed reorganising and developing maternity services to meet the needs of the most vulnerable women in the community, to help them to access services more easily and without judgment.

There is a vast amount of evidence that demonstrates that the more economically deprived or socially isolated an individual is, the more likely he or she is to have poor health. This means that to achieve the same health outcome for vulnerable women as for those who are in a more comfortable position, midwives and other health care workers may need to provide a greater input.

My role was to aim to lead an agenda in which not only the services themselves adapted and changed, but also the staff were made more aware of health inequalities.

One of the biggest challenges was to influence judgmental attitudes. There was (and still is to some degree) a belief amongst some health professionals that people's poor health is often 'their own fault', and there can be little understanding of social and health inequalities.

During my career I saw how women who were disadvantaged in some way due to their appearance or where they hailed from would often be criticised. Comments were commonplace, from 'It doesn't cost much for soap and water' to 'I'm not judgmental, but she's riffraff'.

When things like this were said privately amongst health workers it is likely that the women they were talking about would have subtly picked up on their attitudes. The potential impact of this is that women and families feel judged, and therefore don't attend appointments.

Consequently I set up training sessions relating to all the public health issues – domestic abuse, teenage pregnancy, drug misuse and mental illness.

I worked with a group of wonderfully motivated midwives who helped me to deliver these sessions and who often led the agenda in trying to influence our service in that area.

I will be forever indebted to these midwives as they helped me enormously and felt as passionately about their work as I did. They went far beyond the call of duty to try to improve care for the women most in need.

It was also my responsibility to engage with individuals from the local communities who used our maternity service, to find out what they thought about us and to obtain their opinion on how we should do things.

Sometimes that meant dealing with complaints of varying kinds where I'd listen and, if appropriate, apologise for any mistakes or misunderstandings.

I would always ask the person complaining if they had any ideas how we could do things differently and also invite them to come into the service and show us or to be part of the solution. Sometimes this led to far-reaching consequences.

One such complaint came from an angry grandmother, Marilyn, who wrote to highlight the inadequate care she felt her daughter had received on one of our wards.

I called Marilyn and made an appointment to see her at her home. Over a cup of tea Marilyn listed the catalogue of grievances she had.

'When my daughter had her baby she was left on the ward and not cleaned properly,' she said, with the distress showing on her face. 'The toilets at the hospital were filthy and she hardly got any hot drinks.'

I could understand why she felt angry so we talked about how things could improve and some of the issues I needed to go back to address and rectify. In a lovely gesture Marilyn offered to come and do some voluntary work at the hospital, giving out drinks on the ward, as she said there didn't seem to be enough support workers for those tasks.

Whilst I understand that not all complaints can be put right by the complainant coming to the hospital to do the job themselves, it gave Marilyn the opportunity to provide us with an outsider's view of how we could improve. Marilyn also got involved in helping us to design our new service, years later. She helped to form a group of mothers and grandmothers who had a vested interest in the development of a larger maternity unit and three birth centres. Her input was invaluable.

Increasing the amount of help we got from voluntary workers had a dual benefit. Not only did it provide midwives and staff with extra support but it also gave women an opportunity to be involved in the health service and to increase their skills and potential job opportunities too.

Some of the women I met had been through difficult times and wanted a change, and they saw volunteering for the NHS – especially maternity services – as a stepping stone to other things.

There are too many brilliant success stories to mention; amazing accounts of women such as Safira, who had never worked in England and wasn't computer literate, but came to volunteer with us.

Safira undertook training in diet and nutrition in pregnancy, then came into the diabetes clinic on a weekly basis to talk to the south Asian mothers with diabetes about how they could improve their diets.

Safira went on to learn computer skills and helped to create an information DVD to be given out to south Asian women who were pregnant. The success wasn't just the end product but the confidence Safira gained and the experience she could add to her CV.

Ever since her stroke Mum had periods where she was ill or sick and would need to be taken to hospital.

Whenever this happened my sisters and I were always there with her because she couldn't speak. We were quite strong-minded about it and very protective.

On one occasion Mum had had a nasty fall and when she was taken to the emergency department at Blackburn I was already in the hospital and able to get there really quickly.

She was being attended to by a brilliant doctor, who was new to the hospital. This doctor had no idea I was a senior manager and I watched, touched, as she cared for Mum so sweetly.

Immediately picking up that Mum couldn't speak, she bent down to look Mum in her eyes.

'Is it OK if I speak to your daughter?' she asked. Mum smiled and nodded. Then as she examined Mum she made an effort to speak first to her then to me.

When she bid Mum goodbye I followed her out the room.

'Can I have a word?' I asked. 'I wanted to tell you what you did just then was amazing. If every doctor could do what you do it would make such a difference.'

As she listened I saw her face crumble and she started to cry.

'No one has ever told me that before,' she said, wiping her tears away with her fingers. 'I've had the most awful day so far. My two children are being really hard work, I fell out with my husband this morning and I nearly had a crash driving to work. Thank you!'

It made me realise that while we tend to be very vocal when we are dissatisfied it is not often that we give positive feedback. When Mum could speak she had always given encouragement to people.

It's important to go about what you're doing in such a way that it makes a difference. The NHS is really struggling and if we just spent more time caring for each other then things would be a lot better.

Part of my role as consultant midwife was to work at the University of Central Lancashire in Preston within the midwifery research department.

Seeing as my post was a joint appointment between them and the maternity hospital at Blackburn it was my job to encourage more midwives to undertake academic research, as historically doctors were the professionals that undertook or participated in academia.

We started small with a couple of midwives who were interested in research and wanted to progress, and we took it from there.

My manager at the university was Professor Soo Downe, the director of the midwifery research unit, who was not only a brilliant academic but also an inspirational mentor for me.

Soo was very helpful in further shaping my career and

was also an enormous support when I was engulfed in the Baby Rose litigation case. She regularly listened to me as I rambled on about the inaccuracies of the allegations and we even asked the solicitors if Soo could look at the case records. As an expert in the field she gave her opinion – she too dismissed categorically the claims against me.

I'd never truly recovered from my character assassination in the local papers and worried deeply about the allegations made against me by the expert witness for the claimant – particularly as she was a senior member of staff at the Royal College of Midwives (RCM).

I had never met this woman but every three months I was invited to meetings at the college in my consultant midwife role. The meetings were held at the RCM main office in London where this midwife worked as part of the senior team and each time I attended I felt increasingly anxious. As soon as I walked through the door I would have a huge knot in my stomach and my adrenaline levels would soar. Was this midwife in the building? What if I saw her?

During a conference there I noticed her name in a report I'd just been handed. Immediately I felt winded as the injustice of the situation came flooding back. I had been a member of the RCM my entire career. Surely, I thought, there was a conflict of interest here? I was and still am a great advocate of the college and had even received professional support when the allegations were printed in the papers. Yet a senior member of the same organisation was an expert witness contesting my practice?

On my return to Blackburn I discussed it with both Mrs

Quinn and my allocated solicitor, who suggested I could inform the college of my concerns.

However, I was also quite wary. I felt uncomfortable complaining and at this time I was so emotionally drained by the whole situation that I had little fight left. I felt anxious about relaying the story of the litigation case from beginning to end to yet another person so I held back.

Then the inevitable happened. One day at the Royal College of Midwives annual conference I was sat in the RCM stand in the exhibition hall waiting for a colleague. I had completely forgotten my plight when suddenly I spotted the name badge of one of the two women walking towards me. There she was, right in front of me, the woman who had been writing pages and pages of negative and damning detail about my practice.

Momentarily I was frozen to the spot but, feeling the tears coming, I got up and rushed through the crowded passageway between the stands and headed for the bathroom. En route I bumped into Pauline, who had just been for a coffee with a friend.

'Sheena, what on earth is the matter?' she asked, chasing after me.

The upshot of this dreaded encounter was that Pauline immediately wrote to the General Secretary of the College and explained the situation. As it happened they were unaware that any of their employees were acting as expert witnesses in obstetric litigation cases and agreed that there was a conflict of interest. From then on, RCM employees were not permitted to act in this role.

In the end the litigation proceedings continued until

2004, when I received a letter from the Trust's solicitors informing me that the claimant (Emma) had withdrawn the case. I later found out from Emma that the reason for this was that she was unhappy with the process, as it didn't reflect reality. The case was eventually settled out of court.

As I held the paperwork in my hands I was visibly shaking. Could this really be the end? Was my ordeal finally over?

It was such a relief to learn that I wouldn't be cross-examined in a high court after all.

Years before, as a supervisor of midwives, I'd accompanied a midwife to court when she was called as a witness for a case involving a baby that had suffered brain damage at birth. Observing the event had been a dreadful experience as I saw eminent health professionals reduced to quaking wrecks by arrogant barristers. The thought of being grilled on the witness stand was a recurring nightmare for me and I'd often have fitful nights' sleep because of it.

But although I felt intense relief, that was where the happiness ended. There was no rejoicing as too much damage had been done. My relationship with Emma and her family had ended, my character had been defamed publicly and, saddest of all, little Rose was still in need of intensive support. The settlement they'd eventually received was small and I knew the family would still be struggling.

I hadn't expected to speak to Emma again, but then in a twist of fate Soo Downe, my friend and colleague, met Emma during a meeting at the university where Soo worked in Preston.

As they chatted about Emma's circumstances, Soo

suddenly realised that she was talking to the mother in the case she had often offered me advice on.

'Was your midwife called Sheena?' she asked.

Emma too was surprised but that chance meeting led to Soo formulating a radical idea. A few months later she asked if Emma and I would consider talking together about our experiences to students and midwives at two separate events.

Just a few weeks later Emma and I met up for the first time at a local countryside pub. As we talked breathlessly about our mutual hell during the legal dispute there were hugs and tears.

'It's been so hard,' Emma said, her eyes filled with sadness. 'It's really good to see you again.'

It pained me to hear how much Emma and her family had suffered over the years and that she was still battling to get adequate help with Rose.

But eventually we got round to talking about Soo's suggestion and began to discuss how we could deliver a session that wouldn't be too traumatic for both of us but would have the desired impact. We agreed to each write an account of what it had been like for us and took it from there.

After the emotional rollercoaster of Emma's litigation case I received a very welcome lift when in 2004 a very posh-looking embossed envelope arrived in the post for me.

When I opened it I couldn't believe my eyes.

'Mr and Mrs Blair invite you to tea,' it read. I literally shrieked with excitement. It said something about services to the community and it seemed I'd been nominated by the Department of Health.

At the time Tony Blair was in the midst of a drive to reduce health inequalities and to improve the lives of those living in social deprivation, something I had also been doing my best to tackle in my role as consultant midwife.

I was delighted to be meeting the PM and also felt it was a clever move on his part to acknowledge the work public sector staff were doing.

Typically the date of the tea party fell on a day that I was on holiday in Spain with my family, but I flew back especially.

I'd bought a new outfit, a brown linen trouser suit, and travelling to Westminster my stomach churned with a mix of excitement and nerves. I read the advice sheet over and over, which noted facts like my bag would be searched and that I couldn't bring a camera. It all added to the excitement.

Arriving at the gates of Downing Street I joined a line of smartly dressed people. We were admitted through the door to Number Ten a few at a time.

When I stepped inside I was amazed by the grandeur of the building but it was the great sense of history that struck me the most. I thought of all the prime ministers who had come before and the important decisions that had been made in the building. It was amazing to be there.

The foyer was huge and welcoming, light cream in colour with beautifully painted cornices on the ceiling, and in front of us there was a sweeping staircase with photos of past PMs on the walls. The staff were friendly and the atmosphere was calm as we waited in the foyer. Eventually we were led into a large room that had adjoining doors into other large rooms where we would mingle. Drinks were passed round, as well as small sandwiches, snacks and tiny cakes.

Then Tony Blair appeared, shaking my hand and making time to talk to a few of us at once. I was surprised by his size as he seemed smaller than I had expected.

I introduced myself and told him I was a consultant midwife working with vulnerable families. He smiled and then shook hands with the next person. After going round to meet everyone he thanked us all for making a difference. He also gave a little talk and we then had photos in a group by a fireplace.

I met some interesting people there, lots of other nurses and health workers and some from social care who were equally starstruck. I felt very proud of the service I worked in that day.

When I stepped outside three hours later, I was met by a beaming Anna and my niece Jane and off we went to celebrate with champagne. Eagerly I described every minute of my little adventure and we toasted the PM!

It was also a lovely opportunity to hear all about Anna's job as a midwife at Guy's and St Thomas' Hospital, which she was loving. It was wonderful to see her making her own mark in the midwife world. Often when I spoke at a conference, young midwives would approach me. 'Are you Anna Byrom's mum?' they'd ask. 'She's lovely, such a brilliant midwife.' I always felt immensely proud.

Unbelievably I was nominated to attend Number Ten

again the same year, this time by the Royal College of Midwives. I couldn't believe it and felt equally overwhelmed. The experience was similar, only this time I sort of knew my way around!

This time I wore a cream dress and although Tony didn't manage to get to the group I was stood with, Cherie spent a while asking each of us about our jobs. She was lovely and ordinary really and talked about her children. I will never forget those wonderful days.

As well as the work we did together at the university, Soo Downe and I were keen to work closely to develop initiatives within the maternity service that would improve the quality of the care women received.

We came up with the idea to have a caseload midwifery team in East Lancashire, where midwives would provide care for the most vulnerable women in the borough – those with mental health problems, child protection issues, or those who had had a previous traumatic birth experience.

The caseload team, managed and led by midwife Anita Fleming, were chosen for their philosophy of birth rather than their years of experience and they worked closely with obstetricians to ensure women with complicated pregnancies got the best possible outcome. They went on to win national awards and are still practising in this way today.

We also worked on a Labour government initiative called Sure Start, set up to promote health and social care for children from prebirth to preschool. The overarching aim of Sure Start was to break the cycle of deprivation and to give young children opportunities, regardless of their background.

At last, health inequalities were being tackled, with a variety of agencies coming together to make an impact on the lives of small children. It was very exciting.

As part of the project we created Sure Start midwifery posts to provide intense support to women who were having problems coping with their pregnancies. These midwives had more time to spend with women and to encourage them to make changes in their lifestyles, during and after the birth.

One such woman was Amanda, who was referred to a Sure Start midwife called Sandra for support when she was about six months' pregnant with her third child.

Amanda had left her first two children after suffering extreme postnatal depression. She believed she was a bad mother who couldn't cope and didn't deserve children. Now she was petrified about being a parent again.

'I'm terrified,' she told Sandra during their first meeting. 'I spend most of my time crying and just can't see how I am going to manage.'

She was worried Sandra might think her crazy and admitted that she was wracked with guilt every day at leaving her first two children.

After their first meeting Sandra was able to support Amanda all the way through her pregnancy and during her early days of being a mum. She also began Cognitive Behavioural Therapy (CBT) for her depression.

To Amanda's amazement she found that this time she

was enjoying being a mother and she also began to see her eldest two children regularly.

With her newfound confidence Amanda even went on to become a volunteer breastfeeding supporter, helping on the wards of the maternity department at Queens Park and then on to paid employment in health care.

Meanwhile in 2005 our family was experiencing wonderful times of our own. My eldest daughter Anna was pregnant with her first baby and Paul and I were very excited by the prospect of meeting our first grandchild.

Although she'd been living in Southampton, Anna and her boyfriend Shaun moved home to Whalley to be near family as her due date grew closer, and Anna transferred her midwifery care to Blackburn.

I'd asked Anita, the caseload team leader and a friend of mine, if she was willing to be Anna's midwife. She agreed and Anna also asked her cousin Claire (my sister Anne's second child), who worked as a midwife in Blackburn, to be there.

As her due date approached Anna hired a birthing pool as she started to make arrangements for a home birth at ours.

Her pregnancy had been good and I was relieved to see she was nowhere near as sick as I'd been when I'd carried her.

But Anna's pregnancy seemed to last forever and as she approached forty-two weeks (two weeks past her due date) she was asked to consider induction. Anna really didn't want to go down that route but in October when she was forty-three weeks, after much debating, she agreed to a dose of prostin, a drug used to kick-start labour.

Despite my protectiveness I wasn't worried about Anna coping with labour and tried to support her as my mother did with me, sort of matter-of-factly: this is what we do!

The prostin was administered at Blackburn and then Anna said she wanted to go home. This hadn't been done before but Anna's consultant, Mrs Schram, and Anita backed her choice.

Back at our home Anna's labour began and her contractions increased steadily throughout the evening. Anna and Shaun had set up the pool in the kitchen, which was candlelit and cosy, and Anna was working well through her labour with support from Shaun and her midwives Anita and Claire.

Keeping a backseat, I busied myself making hot drinks for the midwives and popped in and out to chat to Anna, who was doing really well and coping admirably. When the contractions came she was moving with them, back and forth in the water. I was happy to be in the background and it was also very special to be on the sidelines witnessing my daughter's journey to meet her first baby.

I think my youngest daughter Olivia, still a teenager, retreated to the bedroom not really knowing what to make of things. But apart from a mild moment of drama when Paul had to dash off to the hospital to get Anna more gas and air, everything appeared to be going well.

However, during the early hours of the next day it became apparent that Anna's baby's head wasn't descending properly. Anna's labour wasn't progressing, and after chatting to Anna, Anita and Claire decided to transfer her to hospital. Worried, I called Mrs Schram at home, as she had offered to help if there was a problem, and told her that an ambulance was on its way to take Anna to Blackburn.

'I'll meet you there,' she said. I felt instantly relieved.

So Anna was transferred by ambulance and was seen by Mrs Schram. She confirmed that the baby's head was stuck and wasn't descending and by now there was meconium in the liquor, which can indicate that the baby was distressed.

Discussing the situation with Anna and Shaun it was agreed that Anna's baby should be delivered by Caesarean section.

Anna was given an epidural while preparations were made and also that so that she could be awake during the birth and – bewildered and a little disappointed as she had really wanted a normal birth – she headed off to theatre. Shaun and I also went into the room to be with Anna. I held my breath as Mrs Schram worked her magic. Within minutes Anna's baby had been delivered – a big baby boy who she named Seamus, after my father.

We all cried with relief. One of the greatest highlights in my life has been seeing my daughters become mothers to their children. Anna paved the way and the emotion I felt when I saw her look at her new baby son was indescribable. I believe at that moment daughters suddenly understand what their mothers have felt for their whole lifetime, and for me that was a special moment.

Anna, Shaun and our gorgeous grandson stayed with us for a while before heading off back to their home in Southampton. To this day Paul and I have a very special bond with Seamus.

The following month I celebrated my fiftieth birthday and the women and girls of the family decided to hold a Red Tent weekend (based on the theme of the book by Anita Diamont) in a large, old house in a Yorkshire village.

It was amazing. Each female had to be related by blood, and a direct descendant of my grandmother, Gertrude. There were twenty-four of us altogether and two newborn babies, Seamus, Anna's son, and Thomas, my second cousin Hannah's son. The two new mums shared a room and spent the nights chatting whilst breastfeeding their baby boys.

Some family came from as far as America and we spent the week talking and reminiscing about bygone days. It was wonderful.

During the weekend we all had to share a skill with another relative, such as knitting or hair braiding or simply entertaining them. I made each person a book with their name and photo on the front and I included details of where they were placed in our family. The books were passed around to each relative there and we would write something positive about their owners in them.

The whole weekend was filled with laughter and love – and of course birthing, mothering, mothers and babies were the main topics of conversation.

My niece, Cathy, was going to be forty the month after, in December, and as Cathy had lost her mum Lynne we made her a film about her life. We all watched it together, remembering and missing our beloved sister, friend, mother and aunty.

*

During my career I had at times met women who were very unhappy with their birth experience, but yet there often seemed to be no aftercare to support them. The consequence of a traumatic birth was not only that women could be psychologically or physically damaged, but also there was an increased risk of lack of bonding between the mother and baby.

During one of the early meetings I attended as a consultant midwife at the RCM in London, I met Jackie Dunkerley-Bent who worked at Guy's and St Thomas' in London.

Jackie, an experienced consultant midwife, mentioned a clinic she ran for women who reported having a traumatic birth, or who requested a vaginal birth after a Caesarean section.

She told me that the work had been a huge success and women had benefited from having the extra support and guidance.

'It's amazing how much it helps the women,' she told me. 'It can turn their lives around.'

Speaking to her inspired me to introduce something similar back at Queens Park. I remembered Dawn, the woman who'd been so upset after she felt a Caesarean section had been forced upon her. Talking to her, explaining everything and properly preparing her for her next birth had worked wonders. I was sure there were lots of other women who could be helped in this way.

Back in Lancashire I put together a proposal to set up a referral system so that I would meet with traumatised women and try to help them by listening to their experiences and going through their case notes. There was certainly a need for it and before long I was receiving referrals from midwives, obstetrician health visitors and the GPs of women who felt they had been badly affected by their birth experience.

The mothers were usually pregnant with their next child and dreading the thought of giving birth again. Others had confided in their health visitor after the birth when they realised they were having difficulty connecting with their baby.

Each referral would be received by my secretary, Dawn, who in her usual kind, empathetic manner, would ring the woman and ask if they wanted to meet with me – either at their home, the hospital or somewhere else. Women could either come alone, with their partner or with another relative such as their mum.

During the meeting I would sit and listen to accounts of their birth and with their consent make notes. Recalling the trauma was distressing for them and boxes of tissues and cups of tea were always on hand. Then together we would go through their case record to see what events were recorded.

Sometimes this was enough for women to feel instantly better.

'I didn't know that had happened,' they often said.

'So it wasn't my fault!' was another common reaction. Sadly often women blamed themselves for events that unfolded and had been fixating on that very issue since their baby was born.

Other women would categorically dispute the record,

clearly stating a certain event never happened, or that it hadn't occurred the way it had been logged.

In general their trauma was deep-rooted and the impact of events surrounding their baby's birth seemed to be affecting their relationships too. Some women told me with tears in their eyes about how they were unable to have a sexual relationship with their partner and this in turn put a strain on things at home.

In the main, the listening to and discussion of events seemed to be a positive step. Then, if the woman was pregnant, I would offer them extra help from the caseload team of midwives who would provide one-to-one care throughout pregnancy, labour and the postnatal period. I noticed that women were instantly reassured when this service was offered and the feedback was always excellent.

Chapter 14

Sat in front of me gripping a tissue, Nicola, thirteen weeks' pregnant and very distressed, began to tell me how she was still reeling from the effects of her first child's birth.

As she recounted the story she recalled in painstaking detail the words used by her carers at the time, including careless comments that rendered her speechless. Although Nicola could still feel the environment and remember the smells and the faces like it was yesterday, it was the way she had been spoken to that had instigated the feelings of helplessness and despair.

Her plight had begun with her being given an epidural anaesthetic that rendered her bed bound for her labour.

'You are still only five centimetres dilated,' the midwife had told her, after hours and hours of labour. 'There's no progress.'

Later on when Nicola couldn't push her baby out, the same midwife, with a doctor present, said, 'Your baby is stuck and not moving. We need to get it out.'

Scared and bewildered, Nicola thought it was her fault. She hadn't done it right, and now her baby was in danger.

Nicola's baby girl had been delivered by the doctor shortly afterwards, with the assistance of ventouse.

Not only did Nicola feel that her baby had been 'extracted' but in the process she had suffered a bad tear that caused her numerous problems for years. Being stitched up had added yet another trauma as she remembered how the doctor hadn't uttered a word to her but instead held a conversation with the midwife in the room.

Still suffering from the psychological effects of her daughter's birth, Nicola couldn't come to terms with her latest pregnancy and was absolutely petrified to think another labour and delivery was looming ahead.

'It's making me ill,' she told me, her eyes filling with tears. 'It's affecting my relationship with my family, especially my husband, and I have nightmares and flashbacks. I'm just living in terror at the thought of going through it all again.'

Spending time listening to these mothers also had a huge impact on me. I had never sat and listened to women for so long before, often because of time constraints within my job, and now I felt frustrated that other maternity service staff weren't hearing what these women were saying.

Although the reasons for trauma were different for each individual woman, several themes emerged during the six years that I ran these sessions.

Surprisingly, very few women reported pain as the cause of their suffering. In fact, it was hardly ever the reason for the post-traumatic distress. The main theme that came out was a loss of control – feeling that they hadn't given birth to their baby themselves and that, like Nicola, it was 'extracted' from them.

Interestingly, almost all the women I saw had been induced or had their labours accelerated, or had been given epidural anaesthesia for pain relief.

Luckily I was in a good position to secure further support for the women if they were pregnant but it did make me think a lot about how I could get the message to maternity service workers to prevent the distress occurring in the first place.

I talked to my consultant obstetrician and midwife colleagues and also to Soo at UCLan and we tried to think of ways we could get staff to consider what really mattered to women.

I went on to run some sessions for health professionals, where I described case studies of times when women had been let down by the service.

Sometimes the women themselves attended the sessions and would explain how it was the little things that mattered most. This made the message very clear and was (and still is) the most powerful way of giving feedback to staff.

In Nicola's case I took time to go though her records, showing her what had been written and offering her a clear explanation of the events. Some of her questions were answered and she felt a little better, but it was clear she needed a plan of support this time, so a referral was made to the caseload team.

I advised that Nicola's needs were based on her previous experience and that the same scenario should be avoided this time. Duly she was allocated to see Anita from the case load team, and a second midwife who would cover her care too. Anita encouraged Nicola to see Mrs Schram when she was thirty-six weeks' pregnant, though she was reluctant at first. I also booked Nicola in to see Mrs Martindale, a consultant obstetrician.

Thankfully in the latter part of my career I met the most inspirational consultant doctors, like Mrs Martindale and Mrs Schram, who would work carefully with women to ensure they felt happy and were well supported. Far removed from the power-driven individuals I described from my early years, these consultant obstetricians (consultants who care for childbearing women) had extra skills that ultimately enhanced the childbirth experience of so many mothers. Their knowledge was and is exemplary, but it was their additional qualities that really made them stand out as exceptional doctors.

Nicola was sent to see Mrs Schram as she was worried about the scar of her tear and wanted some advice, but the kindly consultant further reassured her that the team and other members of staff would try their hardest to ensure that her forthcoming birth was a positive experience.

When Nicola went into labour she stayed in control and was active, moving around the birth room and progressing well. However, disappointment came when her baby's head didn't move downwards as it should, just like in the previous birth. Mrs Martindale was asked to help as she was on delivery suite that day.

Anita explained to Mrs Martindale that Nicola was petrified at having to lie down as it brought back so many memories of being bed bound and helpless last time, Mrs Martindale worked round the situation. After reassuring Nicola and gaining consent, she carefully applied the forceps with Nicola in the standing position. This is extremely unusual, as doctors learn the technique with the woman on the bed and her legs in the lithotomy position (with the feet held up by stirrups that are attached to the bed on poles). But Mrs Martindale manoeuvered the baby's head round the bend with the forceps, and then removed them so that Nicola could push her baby out herself.

The next time I saw Nicola she was full of praise for Mrs Martindale.

'When I saw her on the floor underneath me, I couldn't believe it,' she said. 'The easy option would have been to make me get on the bed, but she did it for me. I will never forget her.'

Knowing Mrs Martindale it didn't surprise me. Having met Nicola she understood her desire not to labour or give birth to her baby on the bed so she had gone out of her way to respect that. Mrs Martindale has an amazing ability to put women's needs before all else, often pushing boundaries and influencing other more junior doctors to do the same. Doing a forceps delivery in this way is unheard of and the midwives were just as thrilled as Nicola to witness it and be part of the occasion.

Joanne was another mother struggling to come to terms with her impending labour who received wonderful care from Mrs Martindale.

Her first son, Francesco, had been born two and a half years earlier by emergency Caesarean section – an ordeal that was not only traumatic but was followed by a painful recovery.

Joanne explained that everything had seemed rushed and complicated and it had been tremendously worrying for her and her husband, Lorenzo. Consequently she did not feel part of Francesco's birth.

'I had no control, no influence and nor could I be of any assistance to my own son's birth,' Joanne recounted later. 'The only positive was that I was awake during it – although I couldn't see anything.'

The fact that Joanne had endured major abdominal surgery as well as labour took its toll and for a substantial period of time all Joanne could remember was a blur of people coming and going with a vague memory of a baby crying.

It transpired that Joanne had been given morphine to help with the pain and so much of Francesco's first twelve hours was a haze to her.

'The next day I couldn't do anything for my baby,' she added. 'I couldn't attend to him, feed him, change him or even cuddle him properly. I was reliant on the midwives to help me and felt utterly useless as a mother.'

Although Joanne had bonded well with Francesco, not being active enough to tend to him quickly meant he would get upset, leaving her guilt-stricken.

Joanne's recovery at home had been slow too. She relied on help from her family and dreaded the day Lorenzo's paternity leave ended.

'Everyone said that it would be difficult and life-changing to have a baby and they weren't wrong!' she concluded. Now pregnant with her second child, Joanne had so many fears and questions about the birth. Would she have to have another section? Could she have a natural birth? What were the risks?

She described how she'd been confused by conflicting

advice from those who preached 'Once a section, always a section', and other C-section mums who'd heard a vaginal natural birth was still possible but didn't want it themselves.

Joanne was adamant that this time she wanted a normal birth in order to be in control, to feel involved and to ensure she could get back on her feet as quickly as possible. Although a consultant had told her she could have a normal birth, Joanne was still anxious about things going wrong.

When she went into labour Joanne's contractions were short and quick but after two hours of pushing she was utterly exhausted and getting desperate. Everyone around her was trying to keep her calm but she was worried that if the baby didn't move she would need another C-section.

With her dreams of a normal delivery fading fast, Mrs Martindale was called in to check on her.

'She told me that I was doing well but that she would gown herself up just in case she could help,' Joanne recalled. 'The mood in the room instantly changed, I felt less desperate and more reassured that I wasn't alone, pushing in vain.'

After yet more pushing, Mrs Martindale told Joanne that she was going to help the baby along with a little suction.

'Not help me, but help Rocco,' Joanne added when she recounted her experience later. 'The very second she said this was the moment that the stress and fear subsided completely. I was still in control but she was just helping because I was tired. I felt positive, like I had just got a new lease of energy and was ready to meet my baby.'

True to her word, Mrs Martindale used the suction to get

the baby past the U-bend where Joanne had been struggling. After she'd pulled Rocco out by about one centimetre she turned the suction off and told Joanne to carry on.

'She didn't take the ending away from me,' said Joanne. 'A little pull was all I needed and I pushed Rocco out myself. I was exhausted but elated. It was a completely different feeling and experience.'

The impact of Mrs Martindale's practice in these two cases was that both women felt that they were in control and that they had given birth to their baby even though they needed a little help.

A few years later I was to learn first hand just how important Mrs Martindale's skills and compassion were.

When my youngest daughter Olivia gave birth to her son Archie in November 2009, Paul and I were in Australia. Being away from her was traumatic in itself, but when Olivia went to the hospital in labour she had all the signs and symptoms of pre-eclampsia: high blood pressure, protein in her urine and her reflexes and blood picture were abnormal. Anna was with her, and Curtis, her partner, but as we were on the other side of the world we were frantic with worry.

The staff on the delivery suite were wonderful. Paula, the shift leader that day, sensitively kept me informed and Janet (my midwife friend from my community days) and Gill cared for Olivia with expert attention, like she was their own family. One of the absolute benefits of being part of such a close-knit team in the health service is the assurance that your colleagues and friends will pull together in times of need.

Mrs Martindale (as Mrs Schram had done with Anna) had told me to call her if there was a problem with Olivia, so when Paula told me Olivia's condition was serious I asked her to call her at home.

'Please ring her as soon as possible,' I pleaded. I heard shortly afterwards that Mrs Martindale had gone to the hospital even though it was her night off and it was her daughter's birthday.

We were overwhelmed with gratitude. Mrs Martindale repeated her 'manoeuvre' on my daughter, assisting Archie's descent with the ventouse, and then she took the cup off and encouraged Olivia to push him out herself.

As a mother and a midwife I could never put into words how I felt when Anna talked to me later about Olivia and Archie's birth. I was very sad to be away from my daughter but with Anna's love, Janet and Gill's special care and Mrs Martindale's wonderful skills both Olivia and Archie were in the best of hands.

It never failed to touch me the way that caring consultants like Mrs Martindale would listen and tailor births completely to the needs and feelings of the women involved.

When women requested a certain type of care that was different to the norm or an alternative to what clinical guidelines suggested then they'd take the time to consider the options.

Then, even if it were not usual practice, they would often assist the midwifery team in putting together a support plan to ensure the best possible outcome.

And this is what eventually happened with Nadine, a health visitor that I'd worked with during my years as a team midwife.

I was sat in my office when Nadine arrived in a very distressed state, mopping her eyes with a tissue.

'Nadine, what's wrong?' I asked, springing up from my desk.

It turned out that Nadine, pregnant with her second child, had just attended the antenatal clinic at the hospital.

She explained that her first baby had been in the breech position before the birth and consequently she'd had an elective Caesarean section. This time the baby was facing the normal way, head down, and she wanted to have a vaginal birth.

'Having a baby this way is really important to me,' she said. 'I've got a bad back and need to be mobile.'

She explained it was already a struggle to pick her child up in the morning without first having a shower to release her back. So her plan was to move around a lot during her labour and use a birthing pool to help her.

She had wanted to run through this with the consultant but he was away on holiday, so instead she was left to explain her plan to a doctor at the clinic.

But this doctor had told her that she couldn't have her birth this way. In his opinion she would be best on a bed, as they would need to monitor the baby's heartbeat continuously with the electronic monitor. According to him, she was 'high risk' due to her previous Caesarean section.

Nadine started to cry as she added that the midwife who'd come in the room had completely backed the doctor up. There was no negotiating. What upset her most of all was the fact that she hadn't really been listened to or had her worries acknowledged.

The solution as I saw it was that Nadine should go and see Mrs Schram, so I got her an appointment for the afternoon. Mrs Schram, as I'd expected, sat and listened to Nadine before giving her opinion. She confirmed that whilst continuous monitoring was advised after a C-section, there were other ways of checking things.

She agreed to give her the green light for a water birth and wrote a care plan in her notes for her colleagues to follow.

When it came to Nadine's labour she actually didn't have time to get in the pool but had a very mobile vaginal birth on the birth mats on the floor instead. Afterwards she was extremely happy and very much indebted to Mrs Schram.

From my perspective too it's always been a great honour to work with consultants of the calibre of Mrs Schram and Mrs Martindale.

Often my job would entail visiting our projects and centres to check that everything was running smoothly and on one such occasion I went to see a group of teenage parents. There, Karen, one of the teenage pregnancy midwives, introduced me to Geraldine, an African asylum seeker.

Geraldine had come to England following atrocities in her country involving her family, and her uncle had helped her to escape to England.

She was now a single parent looking after her newborn son Arnold and was being supported by Karen. A few months later I met Geraldine again when she became involved in training to become a breastfeeding volunteer peer supporter.

At the time she was awaiting a decision from the Home Office about her application for UK residency and she was very fearful that she would be made to go home.

'Can you help me?' she pleaded. I wasn't in a position to do anything, but I spoke to the link health visitor to see what the normal processes were.

I saw Geraldine regularly after that. She got involved in other initiatives and came to the university with me on one occasion to a meeting. She loved it, and rightly or wrongly it was clear she was building her hopes up to stay.

In 2005 I went to Australia to speak at a conference and just before we were due to return home I went to check my emails.

There was one from Geraldine. To my dismay I read that she had been arrested in the night and was being held in a detention centre in Dover.

She was desperate and explained that there was a possibility that she would be released if she could stay with a UK resident willing to sponsor her.

If not, she would be deported back to Africa the following week.

'PLEASE COME FOR ME!' the email read.

I was about to get on the plane back home but, after discussing the options with Paul, I emailed Anna in London and filled her in.

Anna, who's always been a chip off the old block, immediately drove to Dover to get Geraldine and brought her back to our home in Whalley.

Geraldine and Arnold stayed with us for a few weeks and we all got together to try to help her formulate an appeal to stay. Another friend, Elaine, kindly allowed Geraldine and Arnold to stay with her for a while too, but eventually there were no options left for them and they were deported home.

It was a dreadful situation, and whilst I understand the implications of an overpopulated country and the politics of illegal immigration, I got to know this little family as individuals, understood their plight and wanted to help them.

I never heard from Geraldine again and I often wonder how her and Arnold are and whether they've found safety and happiness. I hope they have.

At monthly meetings at the university (UCLan) I often chatted to Soo about how we could improve feedback from women to staff working in maternity services. Soo suggested we met with some of the women who had been to see me regarding their traumatic birth experience. 'Why don't you ask them what they think you should do?' Soo suggested.

So I invited them all to a meeting at a local children's centre in Accrington, and a few weeks later we were sat drinking tea with ten mothers and jotting their ideas on a flip chart. Soo and I had some suggestions too, and when we came up with the idea of developing a piece of theatre acting out scenarios such as an event on the delivery suite, the women thought it was a great idea, although some of the shyer members of the group said they'd prefer to help 'in the wings'.

At the time Anna was part of a midwifery theatre group, Progress Theatre, so I approached the director and manager, Kirsten, to ask if she would be willing to help.

She loved the idea and in no time at all we arranged to introduce Kirsten to the group of mothers during a meeting at my home. Kirsten came up the night before and we went through copies of her thoughts to help and coach the group.

The next morning I waited nervously for the women to arrive.

'What if they don't come?' I said.

I was interrupted by the doorbell. There on my doorstep looking slightly apprehensive was Helen. Then Sarah arrived, swiftly followed by Sarika, Jeanette, Sue, Maria, Nicky and Debbie. Some of them had brought their children, who we sent to play in the other room while Kirsten arranged cushions for them to sit on the kitchen floor.

The morning began well. We drank coffee and ate home-made cakes and we carefully broached the subject of their births. This process was highly charged with emotion and all of us in the room cried at one point during the get-together.

The group needed time and a safe space to talk about their birth journeys, and lots and lots of support and encouragement. Kirsten's coaching involved addressing their innermost fears of performing, calming their anxieties and leading a kind of half-singing, half-shouting activity to exercise their voices.

It was decided that the women's birth stories would be recorded and then merged into a scene from a busy shift on a labour ward, which would be acted out.

The group met regularly and we planned the first performance, which would take place at the Normal Birth Conference in Grange-over-Sands in the Lake District. This was an international research conference held bi-annually and organised by Soo.

The day arrived and the group assembled on the lawn outside the luxury hotel where the conference was held. Dressed all in black they looked every inch the thespians even though they were all incredibly nervous.

But taking to the stage they just came alive, throwing their all into each scene and keeping their audience thoroughly captivated. It was hugely well received and many delegates came up afterwards to say they were stunned by the bravery of the women and the realistic content of the 'play'.

The impact of the group's perfomances was wide and varied, with many maternity care workers reporting that witnessing the play influenced how they practised and others saying that it really made them think. The group went on to perform at various venues around England and even one in Dublin too. Kirsten and I would always try to be at the 'gig' to support the actresses. We had some fabulous, memorable times getting to know each other and formed some everlasting friendships during our time together.

On a couple of occasions if one of the group couldn't make the booking due to other commitments, I had to stand in. This was nerve-wracking to say the least, but it was also hilarious, as playing a pregnant woman in labour whilst in my fifties wasn't easy! The women helped me so much, but they also laughed hard at my acting skills. My daughter Anna joined the group later on and Debbie left as she moved to New Zealand.

After three years the group eventually dispersed and some of the women went on to pursue new careers, stating that the opportunity had given them the confidence to try other things.

In 2007 I received some happy news. Anna, Shaun and Seamus were moving back to the north of England to be near to us, which was wonderful for Paul and me. We got to see Seamus most days and Anna even applied for a post as a midwife at Queens Park. It was a strange feeling having her work in the same unit as me, but great too as I was very proud of her. Claire and Maria, my nieces, both worked as midwives within the maternity service too, and so it was becoming a real family affair!

Life was as busy as ever at home. Paul had taken early retirement and was helping with the running of the home. We had a hectic social life with a great circle of friends who enjoyed walking and cycling and holidaying with us.

I also remained extremely busy in my professional life. In 2009 there was a change in the management team structure within the service and I became head of midwifery. Our service was in the process of a huge reconfiguration and my manager wanted me to take on a greater management responsibility.

Blackburn and Burnley hospitals had 'merged' years before, but the maternity service still functioned from two sites: Queens Park Hospital in Blackburn and the Edith Watson Maternity Unit in Burnley (where I had trained to be a midwife). The new plans involved the closure of the Queens Park Hospital maternity service for births and the development of a large new maternity unit in Burnley.

The new facility, the Lancashire Women and Newborn Centre, was designed for use by women with complicated pregnancies or by those in need or potential need of medical assistance from doctors. Those who wanted an epidural would also be catered for there.

Three new birth centres were part of the plan, too – home-from-home facilities where women could give birth with minimal intervention and where the focus was on the promotion of normal physiological childbirth.

For me, the changes prompted mixed feelings. I was sad that our beloved award-winning and nationally recognised maternity service in Blackburn was closing. But I knew the amalgamation was part of a greater plan that I couldn't influence. Another consideration for me was that if we could develop and run birthing centres for women and families, we could have a greater influence on reducing the Caesarean section rate. And of course, the chance of having birth centres once more (Bramley Meade was like a birth centre) where women could labour in calm surroundings was an exciting prospect.

I was concerned about the increasing level of unnecessary medical interventions in labour, resulting in increased Caesarean section rates and associated morbidity. During the latter part of my career I noticed the increase in women's lack of belief in their ability to give birth without epidural anaesthesia or medical assistance.

The chance for midwives to utilise their skills without the interference of unnecessary equipment was a unique opportunity and one that I believed would help to improve women's experience of birth and provide a renewed energy for the midwives.

In my new role I was embarking on another journey, one of huge responsibility, firstly in helping to secure funding for the Blackburn Birth Centre and then in helping to develop the facility so that it was fit for purpose. All the new venues had to be designed and developed from scratch and, as a team, my colleagues and I worked long and hard for many months, planning and negotiating.

The task of creating the Blackburn facility fell to my colleagues Anita and Caroline who, with their expert skills and passion for normal birth, created a successful centre. Then as part of the service changes I had to prepare all the staff, explaining how the new service would work and why it was important. I worked closely with the management team and the organisation's communications department to develop leaflets and DVDs to inform women and families about the new services.

Then, on a beautiful sunny day in September, the Blackburn Birth Centre was officially opened by Cathy Warwick, the current General Secretary of the RCM.

We marked the occasion with a garden party and by planting a tree symbolising new life. We deliberately decided to invite footballers from the rival teams (Blackburn and Burnley) as it was symbolic of the combining of services for the two towns. The newspapers liked that too!

From the outset the birth centre was a roaring success and so far there have been more than 700 births there in less than a year.

As head of midwifery most of my time was taken up

attending meetings, writing reports and communicating with other members of the team. Unfortunately this meant there were fewer opportunities to meet with women and families.

It was a great pleasure then, when one morning I was contacted by a lady called Mrs Trainer, who told me the company she worked for had raised £300 doing a sponsored car wash.

The money was to be donated to our service and had been raised in memory of baby Ellis, her beloved grandson, who had been stillborn.

It was always an awful experience to hear about a baby that has died – whether it happens before, during or after the birth it is every mother and father's worst nightmare and probably the one thing that couples fear the most during pregnancy. Nothing in the world can prepare expectant parents for the utter shock and despair that follows such an event.

When I was working as a 'hands-on' midwife I was involved in caring for women and their families during times of bereavement. It was heartbreaking to see the anguish parents went through at this time and never something a midwife got used to.

I was deeply touched by Mrs Trainer's openness and generosity and I asked her if she would like me to collect the money from her. I also asked how her daughter and son-in-law were.

'They are still obviously very sad,' she explained. 'In fact, I am worried about them.'

I asked if she thought it would be useful for me to talk to

them and the following week it was arranged that I would visit them at home.

In one of the most memorable meetings of my career, Nadia and Paul were incredible in the way they described the birth and the death of their baby. They gave me an insight into their feelings surrounding their tragic loss, and showed me photos and a film of Ellis, his clothes, his memory box and the bedroom that he never slept in.

One thing that really struck me was Nadia and Paul's ability to grieve together, their closeness as a couple and the support they gave each other. Whilst they were obviously devastated and were still finding it hard to come to terms with, they had spent precious time with Ellis following his birth, and the wider family too had come to the hospital to spend time with him.

I remember thinking how different this situation was to when I started as a midwife, when there wasn't the same understanding of the importance of offering bereaved parents time with their little one, and supporting them in their decision.

I also thought of my wonderful late mother-in-law, Marie. My husband Paul is one of four boys, but Marie's first baby, a girl, was stillborn. Marie used to tell me regularly about Rosemary, her only daughter. Marie was newly married when she found out she was pregnant and both she and Norman, Paul's dad, were over the moon.

Tragically, when Marie was thirty-nine weeks' pregnant she went into labour and was rushed to the hospital. Shortly afterwards it was discovered that there was no foetal heartbeat. Marie told me regularly, 'The midwives and doctors didn't say anything. I could tell by their faces.' With tears in her eyes she described how, 'They put a cross on my stomach where the heartbeat had been heard last. Then one doctor told me I needed an anaesthetic as the baby was dead and they needed to get it out.'

Marie added that Norman wasn't with her at this stage and she felt frightened and sad. When she woke up both Norman and her mother were by her side but had been instructed not to mention the baby.

'There was no baby for me to hold,' Marie said sadly. 'I could hear babies crying in the other ward and I felt sore, but there was no baby. My mother and Norman didn't say anything, they just held my hand and told me I would be all right.'

Afterwards Marie had a long period of stay in Queens Park and would often walk past the ward where she knew the birth had taken place. But there was no closure for her. With no grave, no memento of Rosemary's life and no image of her face, Marie had no solace.

When I asked Nadia and Paul how they had found our service and whether or not there were things that could be improved upon, their feedback was positive. However, they felt that information for parents of stillborn babies was still lacking and said they wanted to help in some way.

They knew another couple who had lost their baby too and said they felt that the support from others in a similar situation was invaluable. So at that first meeting we set about planning some improvements. Paul and Nadia then met up with their friends and decided to develop a leaflet for parents who find themselves in a similar position, giving details of support. Another local mum who had also lost her baby, Kate, got involved too and provided advice on the final version of the leaflet.

In addition, Nadia and Paul came up with the idea to develop small boxes to give to parents following a bereavement, containing small useful items such as a disposable camera, a Babygro and a clay mould to make a print of the baby's feet and hands. The couple's ideas were accepted gratefully and they set about lovingly making up the boxes by hand.

'It helps us when we help others,' Paul told me. 'We are doing it for Ellis.' This service still continues, and the couple and their family amazingly continue to raise funds to finance the boxes to this day.

I am still in touch with Nadia and Paul, and I recently visited Ellis's grave with them, and spent more time listening to their tales of love and loss.

Even though I have been a midwife for more than thirty-five years, this young couple taught me so much. They gave me a greater insight into the grief of parents, and when I am with them I am reminded of the phrase, 'Where there is a heart, there is hope.'

In March 2010, the moment my sisters and I had dreaded came. Our lovely mum passed away, aged eighty-nine.

Mum had been living in a wonderful residence called Abbeyfield in Clitheroe but had sadly been going gradually downhill for some time. She had really struggled for many years with her physical ability worsening as she got older. Yet she battled on and never complained unless there was a real problem.

Mum hadn't spoken for more than two decades. She could read but couldn't communicate except with her wonderful eyes.

So explaining that she wasn't well was frustrating for her, and although we learned the cues we all felt desperate when she started to deteriorate.

Thankfully she had wonderful carers and amazing family doctors. Even without her voice, Mum endeared herself to everyone she met and they seemed to grow attached to her loving nature.

She would lift up her good arm when we arrived to see her and shout in pleasure and her grin would light up the room. Her heart was full of love.

Because she couldn't talk, many of the carers used to go and sit with her and tell her their innermost secrets or troubles. And if Mum cried, they would cry too. We knew who the kind ones were, and we will never forget them.

When Mum became ill with dreadful pains in her legs amongst other problems, her GP, Dr Flatley, admitted her to hospital. My sisters and I went with her in the ambulance. She was conscious and held us tight.

The care Mum received in Blackburn was impeccable. The ward was busy and full, but the nurses and doctors made sure Mum was as comfortable as she could be.

After a week Mum was clearly deteriorating and we asked if she could be transferred nearer home, to be cared for at Clitheroe community hospital. This was agreed, and it meant that Dr Flatley would be the doctor in charge once more.

From the moment she arrived at Clitheroe the whole

family gathered round – sisters, brothers-in-law, friends, cousins, grandchildren – all to be with Mum. The staff accommodated our demands compassionately as we learned with heavy hearts that Mum wasn't going to pull through. Mum had been slipping in and out of consciousness and her body was failing. We couldn't bear it. As my sisters and I sat and talked to her, trying to be upbeat, it was a struggle not to cry. When I looked over I could see my siblings were welling up too.

We continued to talk to her, telling her we loved her and stroking her face and hands. Denis, my brother-in-law, massaged her feet and Dominic, his son who was particularly close to Mum, sat for hours with her whispering in her ear.

As Mum's last hours came we couldn't help the tears from falling and we marvelled at how she still looked so strong and warrior-like. What a mother.

My sister Anne was with her when she took her last breath.

It was night-time and Eileen and I were just down the road from the hospital, staying in Anne's house. We all rushed back and Dr Flatley joined us almost immediately. We all hugged tightly and, whilst we felt sadder than we'd ever been, we thought of Mum seeing her beloved Lynne once more and our dad.

We all sat round Mum and looked at her. We thought of the love she had given us, the morality and strength to stand up for what we believed in, and the compassion and sense of fun. She was a mum in a million and now she had gone.

After she died Anne and I asked if we could be the ones to lay her out.

Together we washed her, put her in her nightie and

brushed her hair, talking to her all the way through.

It was heartbreaking but we were determined to care for her. The things we learned in our careers have always enabled us to look after our own family and this seemed like the final thing we could do for Mum. I think she would have been proud.

As I struggled to come to terms with the grief of losing Mum, our family was blessed with happy news. Eileen's daughter Francesca, who I had delivered, was pregnant. It was a wonderful boost.

Later when Eileen texted to update me on Francesca's progress during her labour, I reflected on those moments thirty-three years earlier when Francesca had been born.

Then when the message came in the early hours of the morning declaring, 'It's a girl!' I felt an overwhelming surge of happiness for them all. It was very emotional to see history being repeated and to know another generation had been born. It was a very poignant moment for all of us. My sisters, daughters and female cousins always wait in anticipation when one of our brood is birthing and the excitement of seeing a newborn addition to the family never dulls for us.

There was more good news to come. The following year Nadia and Paul revealed they were going to be parents. When Nadia fell pregnant for a second time she was naturally worried about the tragedy of Ellis's death repeating itself, so she sought reassurance from me almost immediately. What a pleasure it was for me to be in a position to be able to offer help.

And I was overjoyed while on holiday in France to receive a text saying that Nadia had given birth to a healthy baby girl.

Being a midwife is so very special. Whatever role you fulfil in the profession it takes you to the very heart of life itself, to the most intimate moments of families.

So the time had come for me to leave my career.

My decision to leave the NHS at fifty-five was not a difficult one. Paul had taken early retirement years before and I wanted to spend more time at home.

Although first and foremost I am a mother, wife, sister, friend and hundreds of other things, my position as a midwife was a vocation.

The work-life balance that is declared as being the secret to a healthy and happy life didn't exist for me. I am afraid to say there was always a blurred line between home and work, but it was my way of life and at times my work engulfed my world.

As I'd got older I was able to enjoy the fruits of my profession and it was wonderful to see the babies that I helped into the world grow into adults – and in some cases, help them to have children too.

There had been a couple of occasions where I was the midwife for women that I had also 'delivered'. Those moments were unique, and for everyone involved it felt as though time had stood still. I will never forget the emotion and privilege.

In the weeks before I left my position as head of midwifery I was informed that I had won a lifetime achievement award organised by the Trust, after being nominated by a colleague. This was a huge honour for me. It was also something I know I could never have achieved without the help of so many other amazing, dedicated individuals who were there to help me along the way in my career.

As my final working day drew to an end I reflected on my life as a nurse and a midwife and was touched by incredible acts of kindness and thoughtfulness: the health care assistant from years before who sent me a lovely letter thanking me, the emotional emails I received and the wonderful colleagues who planned my send-off.

I was thrown no less than three retirement parties and several get-togethers organised by Anita and Annette.

Touchingly Sue and Annette even distributed memory books where my friends and workmates scribbled down meaningful messages that I will keep close to me forever.

As I said my words of farewell I thanked all the mothers, midwives, doctors and colleagues who'd marked my life so positively and whom I would never forget. You know who you are!

In theory I was now retired but my passion for midwifery couldn't stop and as I was considering a new life of grand-parenting, cycling and gardening, in 2010 something caught my eye.

It was an advert to study for a PhD at the University of Nottingham. The position was for a studentship and would be under the supervision of Denis Walsh, a highly respected male midwife and a good friend of mine.

Denis's subject area is normal birth and for my application I had to develop a research proposal for a study related to normal birth – my specialist subject!

I got it and am now well underway! I enjoy studying and from time to time I am invited to do midwifery-related talks.

Anna now works as a midwifery lecturer at the University of Central Lancashire, and is also undertaking a doctorate (PhD) within the same department. It's good for us both to share a common interest and we feel very lucky.

Meanwhile James lives in Holland and is a pianist and singer. He has two children, Minnie and Quentin, and we try to see them as much as we can.

Our third child Tom was a head chef in Leeds and is now in Australia enjoying a working holiday with his girlfriend, Claire.

Olivia, our 'baby', has surprised us all and now lives in a huge farmhouse with her partner Curtis and son Archie and an assortment of animals.

The four grandchildren bring Paul and me much pleasure. I didn't think I would ever love another child as I did my own, but I do!

Apart from the studying, my retirement will be spent enjoying quality time with my family and Paul and I want to travel, to see more of the world and be free not to come back so soon if we don't want to.

I am still involved in several small projects. One particular interest of mine is to use the media to help to get messages to those I want to influence. So Soo Downe and I have helped to produce a film, *Midwives Work*, which has been funded by the Royal College of Midwives.

The film aims to demonstrate how more midwives are needed throughout the world to reduce mortality and improve outcomes for mothers and babies. It will also highlight how midwives need the right education and regulation and that it is essential that all midwives have the right approach – to be kind, caring and empathetic. The film premiered this year in South Africa at the International Congress of Midwives.

I frequently meet women who I cared for while out and about in my hometown. It is always a joy when I am remembered for the part I played in such a special occasion in their lives.

I know that all my midwifery colleagues share that heart-warming feeling when a woman approaches and declares with excitement, 'You were my midwife!' The pleasure never fades and it has always made me feel incredibly humbled and fortunate.

As many of my close colleagues and friends know, I am passionate about the language and words midwives and doctors use. If we say 'patient' we render the healthy pregnant woman sick, and we place her in a position of vulnerability. It's the same with describing what we do. If we say 'delivering' babies it implies that the midwife made it happen. It's a birth not a delivery. Midwives inadvertently take the power away from women if you claim to have done all the work. It is the mother who has all the sweat and toil of labour, pushing out her baby with amazing endurance, for us to 'catch' at the end.

That's why my daughter Anna calls it 'catching babies', and I couldn't agree more.

Acknowledgements

I am indebted to the following people for helping me to complete this book:

Paul, my husband and friend, for his support and encouragement; my children, Anna, Susan, Eileen, and my sister-in-law, Jill Byrom.

Thank you to Pauline, Soo, Carla, Anita and Sue Henry for their inspiration throughout my career. Many thanks to the Royal College of Midwives, and also Emma and all the mothers who kindly allowed me to share their stories.

To all the staff at Headline, including Carly Cook, Jo Whitford, Patrick Insole and Emily Furniss, and also to my literary agent, Rowan Lawton.

A special thank you to my ghostwriter and new 'mate', Charlotte Ward. What an experience we've had!